World Review of Nutrition and Dietetics

Vol. 117

Series Editor

Berthold Koletzko Munich

Nutrition and Growth
Yearbook 2018

Volume Editors

Berthold Koletzko Munich
Raanan Shamir Petach Tikva/Tel Aviv
Dominique Turck Lille
Moshe Phillip Petach Tikva/Tel Aviv

2018

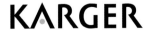 Basel · Freiburg · Paris · London · New York · Chennai · New Delhi ·
Bangkok · Beijing · Shanghai · Tokyo · Kuala Lumpur · Singapore · Sydney

Berthold Koletzko
Div. Metabolic and Nutritional Medicine
Dr. von Hauner Children's Hospital
Univ. of Munich Medical Centre –
Klinikum d. Univ. München
Munich
Germany

Dominique Turck
Division of Gastroenterology
Hepatology and Nutrition
Department of Pediatrics
Jeanne de Flandre Children's Hospital;
and Lille University Faculty of Medicine
INSERM U995
Lille
France

Raanan Shamir
Institute of Gastroenterology
Nutrition and Liver Diseases
Schneider Children's Medical Center of Israel
Clalit Health Services
Petach Tikva, Israel;
and Sackler School of Medicine
Tel Aviv University
Tel Aviv
Israel

Moshe Phillip
Jesse Z. and Sara Lea Shafer Institute of
Endocrinology and Diabetes
National Center for Childhood Diabetes
Schneider Children's Medical Center of Israel
Petach Tikva, Israel;
and Sackler Faculty of Medicine
Tel Aviv University
Tel Aviv
Israel

Bibliographic Indices. This publication is listed in bibliographic services, including Current Contents® and PubMed/MEDLINE.

Disclaimer. The statements, opinions and data contained in this publication are solely those of the individual authors and contributors and not of the publisher and the editor(s). The appearance of advertisements in the book is not a warranty, endorsement, or approval of the products or services advertised or of their effectiveness, quality or safety. The publisher and the editor(s) disclaim responsibility for any injury to persons or property resulting from any ideas, methods, instructions or products referred to in the content or advertisements.

Drug Dosage. The authors and the publisher have exerted every effort to ensure that drug selection and dosage set forth in this text are in accord with current recommendations and practice at the time of publication. However, in view of ongoing research, changes in government regulations, and the constant flow of information relating to drug therapy and drug reactions, the reader is urged to check the package insert for each drug for any change in indications and dosage and for added warnings and precautions. This is particularly important when the recommended agent is a new and/or infrequently employed drug.

© Copyright 2018 by S. Karger AG, P.O. Box, CH–4009 Basel (Switzerland)
www.karger.com
Printed on acid-free and non-aging paper (ISO 9706)
ISSN 0084–2230
e-ISSN 1662–3975
ISBN 978–3–318–06304–2
e-ISBN 978–3–318–06305–9

Contents

List of Contributors

Carlo Agostoni
Pediatric Clinic
Department of Clinical Sciences and
Community Health, University of Milan
Fondazione IRCCS Cà Granda Ospedale
Maggiore Policlinico
IT–20122 Milan (Italy)
E-Mail: carlo.agostoni@unimi.it

Silvia Bettocchi
Pediatric Clinic
Department of Clinical Sciences and
Community Health. University of Milan
Fondazione IRCCS Cà Granda Ospedale
Maggiore Policlinico
IT–20122 Milan (Italy)
E-Mail: pilla.sma@gmail.com

Zulfiqar A. Bhutta
The Hospital for Sick Children
Research Centre for Global Child Health
University of Toronto
Department of Nutritional Sciences
Division of Women and Child Health
Aga Khan University, Karachi (Pakistan)
E-Mail: zulfiqar.bhutta@aku.edu or
zulfiqar.bhutta@sickkids.ca

Kamilla G. Eriksen
Department of Nutrition, Experience and Sports
University of Copenhagen
DK–1958 Frederiksberg, Copenhagen (Denmark)
E-Mail: kge@nexs.ku.dk

Naama Fisch Shvalb
Jesse Z. and Sara Lea Shafer Institute of
Endocrinology and Diabetes,
National Center for Childhood Diabetes
Schneider Children's Medical Center of Israel
Petach Tikva, (Israel)
E-Mail: nammaf@clalit.org.il

Adda Grimberg
Pediatric Endocrinology and Diabetes
The Children's Hospital of Philadelphia
34th Street and Civic Center Blvd.
Philadelphia, PA 19104-4399 (USA)
E-Mail: grimberg@email.chop.edu

Corina Hartman
Pediatric Gastroenterology Unit
Lady Davis Carmel Medical Center
7 Michal Street
34362 Haifa (Israel)
E-Mail: CorinaH@clalit.org.il

Colin Hawkes
Division of Endocrinology/Diabetes
The Children's Hospital of Philadelphia
Philadelphia, PA 19104 (USA)
E-Mail: cphawkes@gmail.com

Liran Hiersch
Department of Obstetrics and Gynecology
Lis Maternity Hospital
Tel Aviv Medical Center, Tel Aviv (Israel);
and Sackler Faculty of Medicine
Tel Aviv University
39040 Tel Aviv (Israel)
E-Mail: lirhir@gmail.com

Anni Larnkjær
Department of Nutrition, Exercise and Sports
University of Copenhagen
Rolighedsvej 30
DK–1958 Frederiksberg C (Denmark)
E-Mail: ala@nexs.ku.dk

Mads V. Lind
Department of Nutrition, Exercise and Sports
University of Copenhagen
Rolighedsvej 30
DK-1958 Frederiksberg C (Denmark)
E-Mail: madslind@nexs.ku.dk

Kim F. Michaelson
Department of Nutrition, Exercise and Sports
University of Copenhagen
Rolighedsvej 30
DK–1958 Frederiksberg C (Denmark)
E-Mail: kfm@nexs.ku.dk

Christian Mølgaard
Department of Nutrition, Exercise and Sports
University of Copenhagen
Rolighedsvej 30
DK–1958 Frederiksberg C (Denmark)
E-Mail: cm@nexs.ku.dk

Luis A. Moreno
GENUD (Growth, Exercise, Nutrition, and
Development) Research
University School of Health Sciences
University of Zaragoza
ES–50009 Zaragoza (Spain)
E-Mail: lmoreno@unizar.es

Moshe Phillip
The Jesse Z. and Sara Lea Shafer Institute
of Endocrinology and Diabetes,
National Center for Childhood Diabetes
Schneider Children's Medical Center of Israel
Petach Tikva (Israel);
and Sackler Faculty of Medicine,
Tel Aviv University, 39040 Tel Aviv (Israel)
E-Mail: mosheph@post.tau.ac.il

Andrew M. Prentice
MRC Unit The Gambia, Banjul, Gambia; and
MRC International Nutrition Group,
London School of Hygiene & Tropical Medicine,
Keppel Street, London WC1E 7HT (UK)
E-Mail: Andrew.Prentice@lshtm.ac.uk

Shlomit Shalitin
The Jesse Z. and Sara Lea Shafer Institute
of Endocrinology and Diabetes,
National Center for Childhood Diabetes
Schneider Children's Medical Center of Israel
Petach Tikva (Israel);
and Sackler Faculty of Medicine,
Tel Aviv University, 39040 Tel Aviv (Israel)
E-Mail: Shlomits2@clalit.org.il

Raanan Shamir
Institute of Gastroenterology, Nutrition and
Liver Diseases
Schneider Children's Medical Center of Israel
Clalit Health Services
Petach Tikva (Israel);
and Sackler School of Medicine
Tel Aviv University
39040 Tel Aviv (Israel)
E-Mail: RaananS@clalit.org.il

Dominique Turck
Division of Gastroenterology, Hepatology and
Nutrition
Department of Pediatrics
Jeanne de Flandre Children's Hospital;
and Lille University Faculty of Medicine
INSERM U995
Avenue Eugène Avinée
FR–59037 Lille Cedex (France)
E-Mail: Dominique.TURCK@CHRU-LILLE.FR

Johannes B. van Goudoever
Department of Pediatrics and
Emma Children's Hospital-AMC
VU University Center
Meibergdreef 9
NL–1105 AZ Amsterdam (The Netherlands)
E-Mail: h.vangoudoever@amc.nl

Michal Yackobovitz-Gavan
The Jesse Z. and Sara Lea Shafer Institute
of Endocrinology and Diabetes,
National Center for Childhood Diabetes
Schneider Children's Medical Center of Israel
14 Kaplan Street
4920235 Petach Tikva (Israel)
E-Mail: MichalY@clalit.org.il

Yariv Yogev
Department of Obstetrics and Gynecology
Lis Maternity Hospital
Tel Aviv Medical Center, Tel Aviv (Israel);
and Sackler Faculty of Medicine
Tel Aviv University
39040 Tel Aviv (Israel)
E-Mail: yarivy@tlvmc.gov.il

Preface

What do neonates, infants, children, and adolescents do that we, as adults, don't do anymore? They grow! Assessing the adequacy of growth in a child is in the DNA of all health professionals involved in pediatric care. And what is (among other parameters) indispensable to children in order to achieve optimal growth? They need to fulfill their nutritional requirements, thereby allowing them to have an optimal nutritional status.

This fourth Year Book on Nutrition and Growth is based on articles published from 1 July 2016 to 30 June 2017. It is the hope of the editors that the summary of the manuscripts and the comments from the reviewers will stimulate the interest of health care providers, physicians, nurses, dietitians, scientists, and many more for evidence based medicine (EBM) in the field of pediatric nutrition and growth. By EBM is meant an approach to medical practice intended to optimize decision-making by emphasizing the use of evidence from well-designed and well-conducted research. The time of weak recommendations from "cooking recipes" and "gut feelings" is over. Our patients deserve to be delivered the best possible care. For this, interpersonal skills, empathy and compassion are obviously needed, but they will be meaningful only if, in addition, decision-making is based on strong scientific evidence arising from randomized controlled trials, systematic reviews, and meta-analyses.

Of course, the coverage of the literature on the topic is far from being exhaustive in the Year Book. The literature search was as comprehensive as possible but for obvious reasons choices had to be made. Some of them may be seen as arbitrary and some readers may be frustrated by the absence of comments on papers that they feel are of very high importance. One of the objectives of the Year Book is to increase the readers' appetite for reading papers of high quality, being able, of course, to keep in mind the main messages of the abstract but more importantly to discuss the strengths and weaknesses of the studies. The ultimate objective of the Year Book on Nutrition and Growth is that our readers would not only read the papers published by other investigators but also would like to get involved in elaborating good research protocols and performing well-designed studies that will enhance the knowledge in the field of nutrition and growth and help colleagues worldwide to be more efficient in the everyday care of their patients.

Dominique Turck, Lille
Berthold Koletzko, Munich
Raanan Shamir, Petach Tikva/Tel Aviv
Moshe Phillip, Petach Tikva/Tel Aviv

Koletzko B, Shamir R, Turck D, Phillip M (eds): Nutrition and Growth: Yearbook 2018.
World Rev Nutr Diet. Basel, Karger, 2018, vol 117, pp 1–14 (DOI: 10.1159/000484497)

The Physiology and Mechanism of Growth

Adda Grimberg[1,2] · Colin Hawkes[1] · Moshe Phillip[3,4]

[1]Division of Endocrinology/Diabetes, The Children's Hospital of Philadelphia, and [2]Department of Pediatrics, Perelman School of Medicine, University of Pennsylvania, Philadelphia, PA, USA; [3]The Jesse Z. and Sara Lea Shafer Institute for Endocrinology and Diabetes, National Center for Childhood Diabetes, Schneider Children's Medical Center of Israel, Petach Tikva, and [4]Sackler Faculty of Medicine, Tel Aviv University, Tel Aviv, Israel

For this year's yearbook, we selected papers related to growth physiology that would be helpful to practicing clinicians. They illustrate the broad range of influences on and variations in child growth. Some highlight the specific nutritional factors of non-cow milk beverage consumption by children and protein-specific effects on skeletal development in a rat model. Others looked at the growth hormone (GH) system, ranging from diagnostic and pathologic issues to non-height effects of growth hormone treatment. Another group explored the other side of the more commonly seen short stature spectrum: a variant of early puberty, a genetic cause of short stature that is associated with acceleration not deceleration of skeletal maturity (bone age), and an up-to-date review of the differential diagnoses and treatment of excessive tall stature. This is certainly not a comprehensive collection of all papers published in the past year on growth physiology and underlying mechanisms, but we hope it sufficiently highlights the nuances and richness of the field to inspire readers to explore the literature on their own.

Key articles reviewed for this chapter

Association between non-cow milk beverage consumption and childhood height

Morency ME, Birken CS, Lebovic G, Chen Y, L'Abbé M, Lee GJ, Maguire JL; the TARGet Kids! Collaboration

Am J Clin Nutr 2017;106:597–602

Skeletal effect of casein and whey protein intake during catch-up growth in young male Sprague-Dawley rats

Masarwi M, Gabet Y, Dolkart O, Brosh T, Shamir R, Phillip M, Gat-Yablonski G

Br J Nutr 2016;116:59–69

Progressive decline in height standard deviation scores in the first 5 years of life distinguished idiopathic growth hormone deficiency from familial short stature and constitutional delay of growth

Rothermel J, Lass N, Toschke C, Reinehr T

Horm Res Paediatr 2016;86:117–125

Reference values for IGF-I serum concentrations: comparison of six immunoassays

Chanson P, Arnoux A, Mavromati M, Brailly-Tabard S, Massart C, Young J, Piketty ML, Souberbielle JC; VARIETE Investigators

J Clin Endocrinol Metab 2016;101:3450–3458

Endocrine long-term follow-up of children with neurofibromatosis type 1 and optic pathway glioma

Sani I, Albanese A

Horm Res Paediatr 2017;87:179–188

The influence of growth hormone treatment on glucose homeostasis in growth hormone-deficient children: a six-year follow-up study

Baronio F, Mazzanti L, Girtler Y, Tamburrino F, Fazzi A, Lupi F, Longhi S, Radetti G

Horm Res Paediatr 2016;86:196–200

Growth hormone positive effects on craniofacial complex in turner syndrome

Juloski J, Dumancic J, Scepan I, Lauc T, Milasin J, Kaic Z, Dumic M, Babic M

Arch Oral Biol 2016;71:10–15

Pubertal progression and reproductive hormones in healthy girls with transient thelarche

Lindhardt Johansen M, Hagen CP, Mieritz MG, Wolthers OD, Heuck C, Petersen JH, Juul A

J Clin Endocrinol Metab 2017;102:1001–1008

Clinical characterization of patients with autosomal dominant short stature due to aggrecan mutations

Gkourogianni A, Andrew M, Tyzinski L, Crocker M, Douglas J, Dunbar N, Fairchild J, Funari MFA, Heath KE, Jorge AAL, Kurtzman T, LaFranchi S, Lalani S, Lebl J, Lin Y, Los E, Newbern D, Nowak C, Olson M, Popovic J, Průhová Š, Elblova L, Quintos JB, Segerlund E, Sentchordi L, Shinawi M, Stattin E-L, Swartz J, del Angel AG, Cuéllar SD, Hosono H, Sanchez-Lara PA, Hwa V, Baron J, Nilsson O, Dauber A

J Clin Endocrinol Metab 2017;102:460–469

Management of endocrine disease: diagnostic and therapeutic approach of tall stature

Albuquerque EV, Scalco RC, Jorge AA

Eur J Endocrinol 2017;176:R339–R353

Association between non-cow milk beverage consumption and childhood height

Morency ME[1, 4], Birken CS[1, 5–7], Lebovic G[2, 4], Chen Y[4], L'Abbé M[1], Lee GJ[4], Maguire JL[1–7]; the TARGet Kids! Collaboration

[1]Department of Nutritional Sciences and [2]Institute for Health Policy Management and Evaluation, University of Toronto, Toronto, Ontario, Canada; [3]Department of Pediatrics and [4]Li Ka Shing Knowledge Institute, St. Michael's Hospital, Toronto, Ontario, Canada; [5]Department of Pediatrics, [6]Division of Pediatric Medicine and the Pediatric Outcomes Research Team, and [7]Child Health Evaluative Sciences, Peter Gilgan Centre for Research and Learning, Hospital for Sick Children, Toronto, Ontario, Canada

Am J Clin Nutr 2017;106:597–602

Background: Many parents believe that non-cow milk like soy and almond milk has health benefit over cow milk. However, non-cow milk has less protein and fat than cow milk and might have, therefore, a different effect on children's height.

Aim: In the present study, the authors sought to determine whether there is an association between non-cow milk consumption and lower height in children and to assess whether cow milk consumption mediates the relation between non-cow milk consumption and height.

Methods: The authors conducted a cross-sectional study of 5,034 healthy Canadian children age 24–72 months who were enrolled in the Applied Research Group for Kids cohort. The primary exposure in their study was the volume of non-cow milk consumption (number of 250 mL cups per day). The primary outcome of the study was height. Multivariant linear regression was used to determine the association between non-cow milk consumption and height. A mediation analysis was conducted to determine whether cow milk consumption mediated the association between non-cow milk consumption and height.

Results: The authors found a dose-dependent association between higher non-cow milk consumption and lower height ($p < 0.0001$). They found that for each daily cup of non-cow milk consumed, children were 0.4 cm shorter. In the mediation analysis, they found that lower cow milk consumption only partially mediated the association between non-cow milk consumption and lower height. They claim that the height differences for child aged 3 years consuming 3 cups non-cow milk/day relative to 3 cups of cow milk/day were 1.5 cm.

Conclusions: The authors concluded that non-cow milk consumption was associated with lower childhood height.

Comments The association between cow milk consumption and height gain was shown in the past in many studies [1, 2]. However, many non-cow milk beverages are produced, marketed and sold in numerous countries in the world as a milk product for children. The present study raises an important issue relevant to many parents all over the world who believe that non-cow milk beverages are better for their children's health. Usually non-cow milk contains less protein than cow milk and does not necessarily contain all the other elements needed to support growth. Indeed, as stated by the authors the USDA MyPlate and Canadian Food Guide have acknowledged that unfortified milk alternatives do not provide the same energy, protein, vitamins or minerals found in cow milk. It is important to stress that it is not just the amount of protein which is important for linear growth but that the source of the protein might have also a crucial contribution to height gain [3]. Despite the fact we know today more than ever what a healthy diet for young children should look like, we still did not figure out the exact mechanism of the interaction between nutrition and growth, especially linear growth. Basic research exploring the mechanism and clinical well-designed prospective studies are needed to produce the ideal growth-supporting diet for the pediatric age group.

Skeletal effect of casein and whey protein intake during catch-up growth in young male Sprague-Dawley rats

Masarwi M[1, 2], Gabet Y[1], Dolkart O[1, 3], Brosh T[4], Shamir R[1, 2, 5], Phillip M[1, 2, 6], Gat-Yablonski G[1, 2, 6]

[1]Sackler Faculty of Medicine, Tel Aviv University, Tel Aviv, Israel; [2]Felsenstein Medical Research Center, Petach Tikva, Israel; [3]Shoulder Unit, Tel Aviv Medical Center, Orthopedic Surgery Division, Tel Aviv, Israel; [4]Biomechanical Laboratory, School of Dental Medicine, Tel Aviv University, Tel Aviv, Israel; [5]Institute for Gastroenterology, Nutrition and Liver Diseases, Schneider Children's Medical Center of Israel, Petach Tikva, Israel; [6]National Center for Childhood Diabetes, The Jesse Z and Sara Lea Shafer Institute for Endocrinology and Diabetes, Schneider Children's Medical Center of Israel, Petach Tikva, Israel

Br J Nutr 2016;116:59–69

Aim: In the present study, the authors aimed to determine whether the type of protein ingested influences the efficacy of catch-up growth and bone quality in fast growing male rats.

Methods: The authors used young male Sprague-Dawley rats who were either fed ad libitum (control group) or subjected to 36 days of 40% food restriction followed by 24 or 40 days of re-feeding with either standard rat chow or iso-energetic, iso-protein diets containing milk protein – casein or whey.

Results: Casein re-fed rats had a significant body weight and longer humerus than whey re-fed rats in the long term. The height of the epiphyseal growth plate in both casein and whey groups was greater than that of rats re-fed normal chow. They also showed that microcomputed tomography demonstrated significant differences in bone microstructure between the casein and the whey groups. Bone quality during catch-up growth depended on the type of protein ingested. The higher epiphyseal growth plate in the casein and whey re-fed-rats suggested a better growth potential with milk-based diets.

Summary: The authors concluded that whey may lead to slower bone growth with reduced weight gain and, as such, may serve to circumvent long-term complications of catch-up growth.

Comments In this article, the authors highlighted an issue that people tend to forget. Not all proteins are alike. The contribution of different consumed proteins to linear growth might be dissimilar even when they are coming from the same source (cow milk in this study). In addition, their contribution to linear growth might not always be directly associated with their contribution to human weight and body mass index (BMI). It is therefore important to study the characteristics of each protein in the diet when height and weight are important, like in the case of growing children.

Progressive decline in height standard deviation scores in the first 5 years of life distinguished idiopathic growth hormone deficiency from familial short stature and constitutional delay of growth

Rothermel J, Lass N, Toschke C, Reinehr T

Department of Pediatric Endocrinology, Diabetes and Nutrition Medicine, Vestische Hospital for Children and Adolescents Datteln, University of Witten/Herdecke, Datteln, Germany

Horm Res Paediatr 2016;86:117–125

Background: Differentiating familial short stature (FSS) and constitutional delay of growth (CDG) from growth hormone deficiency (GHD) and other chronic disease can be a diagnostic challenge. The aim of this study was to determine if growth patterns in the first 5 years of life can be used to differentiate these conditions.

Methods: The authors studied 78 children with short stature (26 FSS, 38 CDG and 14 idiopathic GHD), and reviewed their height standard deviation scores (SDS) in the first 5 years of life.

Results: Height SDS was consistent between birth and 6 months of life, while height SDS decreased significantly after 6 months in GHD, FSS, and CDG. Loss of height SDS was greater in the first 2 years of life than between 2 and 5 years of life in children with CDG (-0.92 vs. -0.11; $p = 0.003$) and FSS (-0.79 vs. -0.01; $p = 0.002$). In idiopathic GHD, the loss of height SDS did not differ between the first 2 years of life and the following 3 years (-0.78 vs. -0.77; $p = 0.821$).

Conclusion: In children with FSS and CDG, there is a decline in height SDS in the first 2 years of life, whereas the height SDS of children with idiopathic GHD decreased almost continuously over the first 5 years of life.

Comments Diagnosing GH deficiency remains a significant challenge, particularly given the poor specificity of stimulation testing [4, 5] and the high prevalence of normal variants of growth among children referred for evaluation of short stature. This study aimed to provide an additional clinical tool to differentiate children over 6 years of age with GH deficiency from FSS or CDG and puberty, namely a detailed review of growth patterns over the first 5 years of life.

The authors showed that reviewing growth trajectories over the first 5 years of life might help to distinguish children with constitutional delay in growth and puberty from those with idiopathic GH deficiency. Maximal reduction in height SDS is seen in the first 2 years of life in children with constitutional delay in growth and puberty whereas children with idiopathic GH deficiency will continue to have a reduction in height over 5 years without this early peak rate of decline. This observation may provide additional reassurance to the clinician observing the growth pattern in a child presumed to have constitutional delay in growth and puberty, hence potentially reducing the number of children undergoing GH stimulation testing.

Reference values for IGF-I serum concentrations: comparison of six immunoassays

Chanson P[1,4], Arnoux A[2], Mavromati M[1], Brailly-Tabard S[3,4], Massart C[5], Young J[1,4], Piketty ML[6], Souberbielle JC[6]; VARIETE Investigators

[1]Service d'Endocrinologie et des Maladies de la Reproduction and Centre de Référence des Maladies Endocriniennes Rares de la Croissance, Le Kremlin-Bicêtre, France; [2]Unité de Recherche Clinique, Le Kremlin-Bicêtre, France; [3]Service de Génétique Moléculaire, Pharmacogénétique et Hormonologie, Assistance Publique-Hôpitaux de Paris, Hôpitaux Universitaires Paris-Sud, Hôpital de Bicêtre, Le Kremlin-Bicêtre, France; [4]Inserm 1185, Fac Med Paris Sud, Université Paris-Saclay, Le Kremlin-Bicêtre, France; [5]Laboratoire d'Hormonologie, Centre Hospitalier Universitaire de Rennes, Centre d'Investigation Clinique Plurithématique, Inserm 1414, Hôpital Pontchaillou, Rennes, France; [6]Service des Explorations Fonctionnelles, Assistance Publique-Hôpitaux de Paris, Hôpital Necker-Enfants Malades, Paris, France

J Clin Endocrinol Metab 2016;101:3450–3458

Background: Different kits for measuring serum concentrations of insulin-like growth factor-I (IGF-I) can give different results for the same sample, despite a 2011 consensus calling for standardization of such assays. This study sought to establish normative data for 6 IGF-I immunoassay kits based on a large random sample of French adults [6].

Methods: Subjects were part of the French VARIETE cohort study, a prospective, national, multicenter, open and nonrandomized study of healthy adult volunteers. A total 972 subjects aged 18–90 years and with a BMI of 19–28 kg/m^2 were considered. After excluding 52 subjects for abnormal values on screening laboratory tests and 11 subjects for missing data on pregnancy status or viral serology, the final 911 subjects (470 males) were stratified by gender and age groups. Serum IGF-I concentrations were measured for each sample by 6 immunoassays and converted to SDS for each technique. Bland-Altman plots assessed pairwise concordance between assays for both raw IGF-I measurements and SDS, and IGF-I SDS were further compared via the percentage of observed agreement and the weighted Kappa coefficient.

Results: Age group and gender-specific normal ranges (2.5–97.5 percentiles) were calculated for each of the 6 immunoassays. The immunoassays shared similar lower limits of the reference ranges, but their upper limits varied markedly. Pairwise concordances were moderate to good with weighted Kappa coefficient for categorized IGF-I SDS ranging 0.38–0.70 and only moderate overall (0.55).

Conclusions: Six immunoassays resulted in different reference intervals for serum IGF-I concentration despite being based on the same healthy population and showed only moderate to good agreement.

Comments Lack of concordance among IGF-I measurements has been considered responsible in part on the reliance on different reference groups for the various tests. Because many factors affect IGF-I levels, the specific inclusion and exclusion criteria defining the "normal" reference group will impact the "normal" reference range values derived from that group. These factors include not just GH action, but age, puberty status in adolescents, gonadal status in adults (e.g., menopausal, on estrogen replacement and whether that replacement is oral or transdermal), nutrition and BMI, renal and hepatic functions, and diabetes status. The sample size of the reference population affects the calculated variance of measurements, and the non-Gaussian distribution of IGF-I values within a healthy population further complicates the calculation of reference ranges. This study demonstrated that differences persist even when different

Grimberg · Hawkes · Phillip

immunoassays are used to measure IGF-I concentrations from the same healthy population.

Lack of concordance among IGF-I measurements is a major problem. Clinicians can misclassify their patients as "normal" or "abnormal" if they compare the IGF-I values measured by their local laboratory against published reference ranges that were measured by a different assay and/or based on a non-representative reference population. Further, results cannot be compared across studies because interassay variability becomes a confounding issue. This has hindered the development of evidence-based practice, and led to calls for standardization or at least harmonization of the various assays. Unfortunately, this problem is not limited to IGF-I [6, 7]; it also plagues measurement of GH [6, 7] and steroid hormone [8] levels.

Endocrine long-term follow-up of children with neurofibromatosis type 1 and optic pathway glioma

Sani I[1, 2], Albanese A[1, 2]

[1]Paediatric Department, Royal Marsden NHS Foundation Trust, Sutton, UK; [2]Paediatric Department, St George's University Hospitals Foundation Trust, London, UK

Horm Res Paediatr 2017;87:179–188

Background: Optic pathway glioma (OPG) is the most common brain tumor (7–20% of cases) that develops in children with neurofibromatosis type 1 (NF1), a multisystem neurocutaneous syndrome affecting 1 in 2,500–3,500 live births. This study sought to elucidate the causative role of tumor location on the development of hypothalamic-pituitary endocrinopathies in children with OPG from NF1.

Methods: Thirty-six children (18 males) with NF1 and OPG (diagnosed by MRI) who did not receive radiotherapy or surgical resection but were evaluated by university hospital endocrine clinics in London between August 1996 and May 2015 were retrospectively followed. Seventeen received only chemotherapy, 3 only decompression procedures, and 2 received both. All 36 received baseline endocrine evaluations at referral and returned every 4–6 months. Dodge criteria classified tumor location as: stage I, optic nerve alone; stage II, optic chiasm with or without optic nerve involvement; and stage III, involvement of the hypothalamus or other adjacent structures.

Results: During a mean follow-up of 9.1 (0.2–13.6) years, 20 (55.6%) children were diagnosed with endocrinopathies. The incidence of endocrinopathies increased with Dodge stage of the OPGs: 0/4 stage I, 12/21 (57%) stage II, and 8/11 (73%) stage III. The first endocrinopathy was found at a mean age of 7.4 (5.0–13.2) years, 2.4 (0–6.7) years after tumor diagnosis. The endocrinopathies diagnosed, in decreasing frequency, were: GHD (36%), central precocious puberty (33%), obesity with insulin resistance/impaired glucose tolerance (11%), early puberty (5.5%), GH excess (5.5%), ACTH deficiency (5.5%), hypogonadotropic hypogonadism (2.7%), and central hypothyroidism (2.7%). GHD was defined as decreased growth velocity over at least 6 months and a peak GH concentration <6.6 µg/L upon stimulation with either insulin tolerance test or glucagon. GH treatment was started in those with stable neuroradiological findings after at least 1 year of monitoring, and of those 13 patients, 9 continued to adult height by the end of the study period while 1 discontinued for worsening of previous severe scoliosis and another discontinued due to tumor progression. All 8 patients whose GH axis was reassessed at adult height had normal GH peaks on retesting.

Conclusions: Children with OPG due to NF1 are at high risk of developing endocrinopathies due to tumor location and thus, warrant lifelong endocrine follow-up.

Comments It is perhaps not surprising to find hypothalamic-pituitary dysfunction to be common among children with OPGs, given the tumor location. What most surprised me in reading this paper was the transient nature of the GH excess. Two of the 36 subjects developed GH excess, defined by tall stature with increased growth velocity, high IGF-I levels, and lack of GH suppression during a 1.75 g/kg oral glucose tolerance test. GH excess was suspected in patients who were prepubertal or whose puberty was clinically and biochemically suppressed by treatment with gonadotropin releasing hormone analog (12 of the 36 subjects with OPGs developed central precocious puberty). The GH excess was suppressed by treatment with a somatostatin analog in both subjects, for 3–4 years. One stopped somatostatin analog therapy after developing acute pancreatitis, and the other upon reaching adult height. Both had normal GH secretion on testing after stopping the somatostatin analog treatment. While less common than GH deficiency among patients with OPGs and NF1 (13 of the 36 subjects in the current study), GH excess has been reported in other studies of patients with OPGs and NF1 [9, 10]. Others have also noted the transient nature of the GH excess [11]. Out of 7 patients with GH excess associated with optic pathway tumors (5 of whom had clinically diagnosed NF1, and all of whom had concurrent central precocious puberty treated with gonadotropin releasing hormone analog), only 3 continued somatostatin analog treatment for an extended period of time, and one was switched to pegvisomant (a GH receptor antagonist) due to somatostatin non-responsiveness. Five of the patients had a resolution of the GH excess with normal growth and IGF-I levels off treatment (the remaining 2 were either never treated or still on treatment at the time of study completion). Thus, this patient population offers a unique opportunity to elucidate the mechanism of the dysregulation leading to transient, excessive GH secretion.

The influence of growth hormone treatment on glucose homeostasis in growth hormone-deficient children: a six-year follow-up study

Baronio F[1], Mazzanti L[1], Girtler Y[2], Tamburrino F[1], Fazzi A[2], Lupi F[2], Longhi S[2], Radetti G[3]

[1]Department of Woman, Child and Urologic Diseases, S. Orsola-Malpighi Hospital, University of Bologna, Bologna, Italy; [2]Department of Paediatrics, Regional Hospital Bolzano, and [3]Marienklinik, Bolzano, Italy

Horm Res Paediatr 2016;86:196–200

Background: GH reduces insulin sensitivity and results in increased insulin secretion. In animal and human studies, it has been suggested that GH might also increase insulin secretion through a direct effect on the growth and function of pancreatic beta-cells. The aim of this study was to describe the insulin sensitivity using the homeostasis model assessment (HOMA-S), insulinogenic index (IGI), and oral disposition index (ODI) in GHD children during GH treatment.
Methods: Ninety-nine children with GHD (62 male, 37 female; age 8.9 ± 3.5 years) were followed for a median of 6 years (range 1.5–16.2). Patients underwent an oral glucose tolerance test annually, and HOMA-S [1/{insulin (mIU/ml) × glucose (mg/dl)}], IGI ($\triangle$ insulin 0–30 min / $\triangle$ glucose 0–30 min), and ODI (HOMA-S × IGI) were calculated.
Results: HOMA-S remained unchanged but an increase in IGI and ODI was observed, which became significant after 6 years of treatment (1.25 ± 1.28 vs. 2.35 ± 2.38, $p < 0.05$ and 0.57 ± 0.68 vs. 1.50 ± 1.92, $p < 0.01$, respectively).
Conclusions: GH treatment is associated with increases in the beta-cell secretory capacity of children with GH deficiency during GH treatment.

Comments   In this 6-year longitudinal study of children with GH deficiency, authors used annual oral glucose tolerance tests to explore the relationship between GH treatment and glucose homeostasis. This study challenges the perception that increased insulin secretion is simply a response to increased insulin resistance. The
IGI was used to describe insulin secretion in these patients, and the authors
showed that GH treatment was associated with increased insulin secretion in excess of that explained by changes in insulin resistance. This work builds on animal
studies demonstrating a trophic effect of GH on pancreatic beta cells [12, 13], and
suggests that this effect may also be clinically detectable in children during GH
treatment.

Growth hormone positive effects on craniofacial complex in Turner syndrome

Juloski J[1], Dumancic J[2, 3], Scepan I[1], Lauc T[4, 5], Milasin J[6], Kaic Z[7, 8], Dumic M[9], Babic M[6]

[1]Department of Orthodontics, School of Dental Medicine, University of Belgrade, Belgrade, Serbia;
[2]Department of Dental Anthropology, School of Dental Medicine, University of Zagreb, Zagreb,
Croatia; [3]Department of Dental Medicine, University Hospital Center Zagreb, Croatia; [4]Department
of Anthropology, Faculty of Social Sciences and Humanities, University of Zagreb, Zagreb, Croatia;
[5]Department of Otorhinolaryngology and Maxillofacial Surgery, Faculty of Medicine, University
of Osijek, Osijek, Croatia; [6]Institute of Biology and Human Genetics, School of Dental Medicine,
University of Belgrade, Belgrade, Serbia; [7]Croatian Dental Chamber, Zagreb, Croatia; [8]Croatian
Academy of Medical Sciences, Zagreb, Croatia; [9]Medical Faculty, University of Zagreb, Croatia

Arch Oral Biol 2016;71:10–15

Background: Mild phenotypic features are seen in the craniofacial region of children and adults
with Turner syndrome. GH treatment is approved in these patients to improve their final height.
The aim of this study was to describe the effect of GH treatment on the craniofacial morphology in
girls with Turner syndrome.
Methods: The authors performed a cross-sectional cephalometric analysis on lateral cephalograms
of patients with 45 X karyotype. They included 13 girls who had received GH for at least 2 years,
and 13 untreated controls who were matched for age and karyotype. Sixteen linear and angular
measurements were taken from standard lateral cephalograms.
Results: The average age of girls included in this study was 17.3 years. In patients treated with GH,
most linear measurements were significantly greater than in untreated patients. GH treatment influenced posterior face height, mandibular ramus height, total mandibular length, anterior face
height, and maxillary length. There was no significant difference in the angular measurements and
facial height ratio. Acromegalic features were not seen.
Conclusions: Long-term GH treatment has positive effects on craniofacial development in patients
with Turner syndrome. The greatest effects are seen on posterior facial height and mandibular ramus. However, GH treatment does not normalize craniofacial features.

Comments   The facial appearance of children with Turner syndrome may include a shorter and
flattened cranial base, retrognathia, and a posteriorly inclined maxilla and mandible.
GH can have effects on craniofacial growth, and this study used a case-control design
to determine if GH treatment has a positive effect on these facial stigmata of Turner
syndrome. The authors have shown that GH treatment may improve these features,
mostly through effects on the mandibular ramus and posterior face height. Although

the craniofacial features did not normalize, the positive effect of GH described in this study provides additional information in discussing the potential pros and cons of GH treatment with these patients.

Pubertal progression and reproductive hormones in healthy girls with transient thelarche

Lindhardt Johansen M[1,2], Hagen CP[1,2], Mieritz MG[1,2], Wolthers OD[3], Heuck C[4], Petersen JH[1,2], Juul A[1,2,5]

[1]Department of Growth and Reproduction, Rigshospitalet, Copenhagen, Denmark; [2]International Center for Research and Research Training in Endocrine Disruption of Male Reproduction and Child Health, University of Copenhagen, Copenhagen, Denmark; [3]Asthma and Allergy Clinic, Children's Clinic Randers, Randers, Denmark; [4]Department of Pediatrics, Aalborg University Hospital, Aalborg, Denmark; [5]Department of Clinical Medicine, Faculty of Health and Medical Sciences, University of Copenhagen, Copenhagen, Denmark

J Clin Endocrinol Metab 2017;102:1001–1008

Background: This study sought to describe transient thelarche (TT), defined as breast bud appearance, regression and then reappearance, after the age of normal puberty (i.e., after age 8 years, as opposed to premature thelarche, which is similar but happens at a younger age).

Methods: This study included 98 healthy Caucasian girls from the longitudinal follow-up of the COPENHAGEN Puberty Study, a public school-based study of healthy children in the Copenhagen area in 2005–2006. Clinical examinations and blood sampling for hormone levels were performed every 6 months 2006–2014, and they were genotyped for FSHR and FSHB.

Results: TT occurred in12 of the 98 girls, but not more than once. The median time from the first to second breast development was 1.47 years (0.88–4.09). More of the girls with TT (50%) started puberty with pubarche, as opposed to 15.4% of the 86 girls without TT. Growth velocity was slower and gonadotropin levels lower with the first (transient) thelarche than the second (permanent) thelarche, and all aspects of pubertal progression associated with the second (permanent) thelarche were normal, resembling those of girls without TT. Neither genotyping (FSHR and FSHB) nor weight/BMI distinguished girls who underwent TT versus those without.

Conclusions: TT is a common, peripheral (i.e., gonadotropin-independent) occurrence independent of central puberty, which progresses normally thereafter.

Comments There are 2 key variables for assessing puberty: age of onset and tempo (how fast a child progresses through the various Tanner stages). Growth ceases at the end of puberty, so both variables play a role. A child can start puberty early, middle, or late and go slow, medium or fast; now add to those various combinations the possibility of TT. This study illustrates the importance of clinically monitoring an adolescent's pubertal development in 6-month intervals to get a feel for their tempo (there are no tests to predict tempo). The risk-benefit considerations of therapeutic intervention (e.g., with a GnRH agonist) may be different for a girl with early thelarche if it turned out to be TT or followed by a slow tempo than if it were compounded by a rapid tempo.

Clinical characterization of patients with autosomal dominant short stature due to aggrecan mutations

Gkourogianni A[1], Andrew M[2], Tyzinski L[2], Crocker M[3], Douglas J[4], Dunbar N[5], Fairchild J[6], Funari MFA[7], Heath KE[8], Jorge AAL[7], Kurtzman T[9], LaFranchi S[10], Lalani S[11], Lebl J[13], Lin Y[12], Los E[10], Newbern D[14], Nowak C[4], Olson M[14], Popovic J[15], Průhová Š[13], Elblova L[13], Quintos JB[16], Segerlund E[1, 17], Sentchordi L[8, 18], Shinawi M[19], Stattin E-L[20], Swartz J[3], del Angel AG[21], Cuéllar SD[21], Hosono H[22], Sanchez-Lara PA[23], Hwa V[2], Baron J[24], Nilsson O[1, 24, 25], Dauber A[2]

[1]Division of Pediatric Endocrinology, Department of Women's and Children's Health, Karolinska Institutet and Karolinska University Hospital, Stockholm, Sweden; [2]Cincinnati Center for Growth Disorders, Division of Endocrinology, Cincinnati Children's Hospital Medical Center, Cincinnati, OH, USA; Divisions of [3]Endocrinology and [4]Genetics, Boston Children's Hospital, Boston, MA, USA; [5]Division of Pediatric Endocrinology, Connecticut Children's Medical Center, Hartford, CT, USA; [6]Department of Endocrinology and Diabetes, Women's and Children's Hospital, North Adelaide, South Australia, Australia; [7]Unidade de Endocrinologia do Desenvolvimento (LIM/42), Disciplina de Endocrinologia, Faculdade de Medicina da Universidade de São Paulo, São Paulo, Brazil; [8]Institute of Medical and Molecular Genetics (INGEMM) and Skeletal Dysplasia Multidisciplinary Unit, Hospital Universitario La Paz, Universidad Autónoma de Madrid, IdiPAZ, and CIBERER, ISCIII, Madrid, Spain; [9]El Rio Community Health Center, Tucson, AZ, USA; [10]Department of Pediatrics, Oregon Health and Science University, Portland, OR, USA; Departments of [11]Molecular and Human Genetics and [12]Pediatric Endocrinology and Metabolism, Baylor College of Medicine, Houston, TX, USA; [13]Department of Pediatrics, Second Faculty of Medicine, Charles University in Prague and University Hospital in Motol, Prague, Czech Republic; [14]Division of Endocrinology, Phoenix Children's Hospital, Phoenix, AZ, USA; [15]Children's Hospital of Pittsburgh, University of Pittsburgh Medical Center, Pittsburgh, PA, USA; [16]Hasbro Children's Hospital, Providence, RI, USA; [17]Sunderby Hospital, Sunderby, Sweden; [18]Department of Pediatrics, Hospital Universitario Infanta Sofia, Madrid, Spain; [19]Division of Genetics, Washington University, St. Louis, MO, USA; [20]Department of Immunology, Genetics and Pathology, Science for Life Laboratory, Uppsala University, Uppsala, Sweden; [21]Laboratorio de Biología Molecular, Departamento de Genética Humana, Instituto Nacional de Pediatría, Insurgentes-Cuicuilco, Coyoacán México; [22]Cottage Children's Medical Center, Santa Barbara, CA, USA; [23]Center for Personalized Medicine, Children's Hospital of Los Angeles, Los Angeles, CA, USA; [24]Section on Growth and Development, Eunice Kennedy Shriver National Institute of Child Health and Human Development, National Institutes of Health, Bethesda, MD, USA; [25]Department of Medical Sciences, Örebro University and University Hospital, Örebro, Sweden

J Clin Endocrinol Metab 2017;102:460–469

Background: Heterozygous mutations in the aggrecan gene (ACAN) are associated with autosomal-dominant short stature and accelerated skeletal maturation. The aim of this study was to describe the phenotypic spectrum and response to growth-promoting therapies in children with heterozygous mutations in the ACAN gene.
Methods: One hundred and three subjects (57 females, 46 males) from 20 families with heterozygous ACAN mutations were identified. Clinical information was collected through chart review.
Results: ACAN variants co-segregated with phenotype. Adults had mildly disproportionate short stature (median [range] height Z-Score –2.8 [–5.9 to –0.9]) and early growth cessation. Early-onset osteoarthritis was seen in 12 families and intervertebral disc disease in 9 families. There was no genotype-phenotype correlation between the type of ACAN mutation and joint disease. Height in children was less affected (median [range] height Z-Score –2.0 [–4.2 to –0.6]) but most children with ACAN mutations had advanced bone age (median [range] bone age – chronologic age; +1.3

years [+0.0 to +3.7 years]). In this study population, 19 patients had received GH treatment with some increased growth velocity.

Conclusions: Heterozygous ACAN mutations are associated with a phenotypic spectrum ranging from mild and proportionate short stature to mild skeletal dysplasia with disproportionate short stature and brachydactyly. Early-onset osteoarthritis and degenerative disc disease is seen in many patients, suggesting dysfunction of the articular cartilage and intervertebral disc cartilage.

Comments  Aggrecan is a proteoglycan that plays an important role in articular and growth plate cartilage matrix and homozygous or missense mutations have been described in cases of skeletal dysplasia with severe short stature and severe joint disease [14–16]. Recently, novel heterozygous mutations in the *ACAN* gene have been identified as a cause of idiopathic short stature and advanced bone age with subtle skeletal abnormalities [17]. This international collaboration expands the phenotype of mutations in this gene through the detailed description of 19 different mutations in 103 subjects from 20 families. A common phenotype in affected individuals is the combination of advanced bone age with early growth cessation. Joint disease was seen in over half of this cohort, mostly presenting before 40 years of age.

Management of endocrine disease: diagnostic and therapeutic approach of tall stature

Albuquerque EV[1], Scalco RC[2], Jorge AA[3]

[1]Unidade de Endocrinologia Genética, Laboratório de Endocrinologia Celular e Molecular (LIM/25), Disciplina de Endocrinologia da Faculdade de Medicina da Universidade de São Paulo, São Paulo, Brazil; [2]Unidade de Endocrinologia do Desenvolvimento,Laboratório de Hormônios e Genética Molecular (LIM/42) do Hospital das Clinicas, Disciplina de Endocrinologia da Faculdade de Medicina da Universidade de São Paulo, São Paulo, Brazil; [3]Disciplina de Endocrinologia da Faculdade de Ciências Médicas da Santa Casa de São Paulo, São Paulo, Brazil

Eur J Endocrinol 2017;176:R339–R353

Background: Patients with tall stature (height above +2 SD for age and gender or more than 2 SD above mid-parental height SDS) are often referred to endocrinologists to exclude hormonal disorders.

Methods: Authors reviewed the differential diagnosis of tall stature and offered a practical diagnostic approach to patients with tall stature. They also discussed the limitations of current growth interrupting treatment options.

Results: The majority of patients with tall stature have familial tall stature or constitutional growth advancement (usually associated with obesity). Both are diagnoses of exclusion. The endocrine causes of tall stature are: GH/IGF-I excess, precocious exposure to sex steroids, prolonged growth due to delayed fusion of the growth plate (hypogonadism, aromatase deficiency, and estrogen resistance), thyrotoxicosis, and obesity. Syndromic causes include: supernumerary sex chromosome aneuploidies and monogenic forms (most notably, Marfan syndrome, Sotos syndrome, Beckwith-Wiedemann syndrome, homocystinuria and Fragile X syndrome).

Conclusions: Advances in genetic testing have revealed a growing list of conditions that can cause tall stature. However, now that sex steroids are no longer widely recommended to cease growth (due to short- and long-term consequences), treatment options are limited; remaining drugs are either of poor efficacy or still considered experimental, and percutaneous epiphysiodesis (surgically attaching the epiphysis and diaphysis of a long bone) is reserved for patients with extreme tall stature >+3 SD.

Comments   The authors' strong background in genetics is evident in this excellent review of multiple conditions that can cause tall stature; not only do they organize the topic by endocrine versus genetic categories of conditions, but they provide a useful table of clinical findings and disorders with which they are associated. Another approach to the topic was taken by Juan Sotos and Jesus Argente in their earlier study [18]. They categorized the differential diagnosis by pathophysiological mechanisms (excess of a growth gene [e.g., *SHOX*]; excess of GH; excess of growth factors [IGF-II, IGF-I, insulin]; excess or mutations of growth factor receptors; deficiency of factors needed to arrest growth [e.g., estrogen]; deficiency of factors needed to prevent bone elongation and dysmorphic proportions; alterations in genes involved in tumor suppression, cell cycle, proliferation and growth; and over-nutrition/obesity). Thus, readers can benefit from 2 excellent reviews of a large, complex topic that complement each other in approach.

References

1 DeBoer MD, Agard HE, Scharf RJ: Milk intake, height and body mass index in preschool children. Arch Dis Child 2015;100:460–465.

2 de Beer H: Dairy products and physical stature: a systematic review and meta-analysis of controlled trials. Econ Hum Biol 2012;10:299–309.

3 Grasgruber P, Sebera M, Hrazdíra E, Cacek J, Kalina T: Major correlates of male height: a study of 105 countries. Econ Hum Biol 2016;21:172–195.

4 Ghigo E, Bellone J, Aimaretti G, Bellone S, Loche S, Cappa M, Bartolotta E, Dammacco F, Camanni F: Reliability of provocative tests to assess growth hormone secretory status. Study in 472 normally growing children. J Clin Endocrinol Metab 1996;81:3323–3327.

5 Marin G, Domene HM, Barnes KM, Blackwell BJ, Cassorla FG, Cutler GB Jr: The effects of estrogen priming and puberty on the growth hormone response to standardized treadmill exercise and arginine-insulin in normal girls and boys. J Clin Endocrinol Metab 1994;79:537–541.

6 Clemmons DR: Consensus statement on the standardization and evaluation of growth hormone and insulin-like growth factor assays. Clin Chem 2011;57:555–559.

7 Grimberg A, DiVall SA, Polychronakos C, Allen DB, Cohen LE, Quintos JB, Rossi WC, Feudtner C, Murad MH; Drug and Therapeutics Committee and Ethics Committee of the Pediatric Endocrine Society; Guidelines for growth hormone and insulin-like growth factor-I treatment in children and adolescents: growth hormone deficiency, idiopathic short stature, and primary insulin-like growth factor-I deficiency. Horm Res Paediatr 2016;86:361–397.

8 Kulle A, Krone N, Holterhus PM, Schuler G, Greaves RF, Juul A, de Rijke YB, Hartmann MF, Saba A, Hiort O, Wudy SA; EU COST Action: Steroid hormone analysis in diagnosis and treatment of DSD: position paper of EU COST Action BM 1303 'DSD-net'. Eur J Endocrinol 2017;176:P1–P9.

9 Cambiaso P, Galassi S, Palmiero M, Mastronuzzi A, Del Bufalo F, Capolino R, Cacchione A, Buonuomo PS, Gonfiantini MV, Bartuli A, Cappa M, Macchiaiolo M: Growth hormone excess in children with neurofibromatosis type-1 and optic glioma. Am J Med Genet 2017;173:2353–2358.

10 Josefson J, Listernick R, Fangusaro JR, Charrow J, Habiby R: Growth hormone excess in children with neurofibromatosis type 1-associated and sporadic optic pathway tumors. J Pediatr 2011;158:433–436.

11 Josefson JL, Listernick R, Charrow J, Habiby RL: Growth hormone excess in children with optic pathway tumors is a transient phenomenon. Horm Res Paediatr 2016;86:35–38.

12 Cordoba-Chacon J, Gahete MD, Pokala NK, Gelder-mann D, Alba M, Salvatori R, Luque RM, Kineman RD: Long- but not short-term adult-onset, isolated GH deficiency in male mice leads to deterioration of β-cell function, which cannot be accounted for by changes in β-cell mass. Endocrinology 2014;155: 726–735.

13 Huang Y, Chang Y: Regulation of pancreatic islet be-ta-cell mass by growth factor and hormone signal-ing. Prog Mol Biol Transl Sci 2014;121:321–349.

14 Stattin EL, Wiklund F, Lindblom K, Onnerfjord P, Jonsson BA, Tegner Y, Sasaki T, Struglics A, Lohm-ander S, Dahl N, Heinegard D, Aspberg A: A mis-sense mutation in the aggrecan C-type lectin domain disrupts extracellular matrix interactions and causes dominant familial osteochondritis dissecans. Am J Hum Genet 2010;86:126–137.

15 Tompson SW, Merriman B, Funari VA, Fresquet M, Lachman RS, Rimoin DL, Nelson SF, Briggs MD, Cohn DH, Krakow D: A recessive skeletal dysplasia, SEMD aggrecan type, results from a missense muta-tion affecting the C-type lectin domain of aggrecan. Am J Hum Genet 2009;84:72–79.

16 Gleghorn L, Ramesar R, Beighton P, Wallis G: A mu-tation in the variable repeat region of the aggrecan gene (AGC1) causes a form of spondyloepiphyseal dysplasia associated with severe, premature osteoar-thritis. Am J Hum Genet 2005;77:484–490.

17 Nilsson O, Guo MH, Dunbar N, Popovic J, Flynn D, Jacobsen C, Lui JC, Hirschhorn JN, Baron J, Dauber A: Short stature, accelerated bone maturation, and early growth cessation due to heterozygous aggrecan mutations. J Clin Endocrinol Metab 2014;99:E1510–E1518.

18 Sotos JF, Argente J: Overgrowth disorders associated with tall stature. Adv Pediatr 2008;55:213–254.

Koletzko B, Shamir R, Turck D, Phillip M (eds): Nutrition and Growth: Yearbook 2018.
World Rev Nutr Diet. Basel, Karger, 2018, vol 117, pp 15–38 (DOI: 10.1159/000484498)

Obesity, Metabolic Syndrome and Nutrition

Shlomit Shalitin[1,2] · Luis A. Moreno[3]

[1]The Jesse Z. and Sara Lea Shafer Institute of Endocrinology and Diabetes, National Center for Childhood Diabetes, Schneider Children's Medical Center of Israel, Petach Tikva, and [2]Sackler Faculty of Medicine, Tel Aviv University, Tel Aviv, Israel; [3]GENUD (Growth, Exercise, Nutrition, and Development) Research, and University School of Health Sciences, University of Zaragoza, Zaragoza, Spain

Childhood obesity is a major worldwide health concern, widely recognized as a risk factor for the development of cardiometabolic comorbidities. Known to affect its occurrence are genetic, environmental, lifestyle, and behavioral factors. Although its prevalence is increasing [1], a recent study reported stabilization of this trend, especially in developed countries [2].

A growing body of evidence suggests that the increased risk for childhood obesity is associated with early-life factors, such as pregnancy weight gain, birth weight, rapid postnatal growth, and gestational diabetes.

In an evaluation of the relationship between breastfeeding during the first 6 months of life and body mass index (BMI) in infancy and subsequent childhood, there were contradictory findings regarding a long-lasting association.

Age at adiposity rebound is a predictor of subsequent changes in BMI pattern, an earlier age being associated with increased risk of overweight. One of the studies assessed the association between breastfeeding and BMI development trajectories from age 2 to 16 years.

Emerging evidence suggests that nutrition during early life may have consequences extending into adulthood. "Early Nutrition", an international research project, has provided up-to-date evidence of the effects of early nutrition on metabolic programming and their consequent health impacts. This report presents current standards, recommendations, guidelines, and regulations on nutrition in healthy term infants and children aged 1–3 years.

Other studies evaluated the associations between dietary intake of fatty acids and fiber during infancy, as well as infant circadian feeding patterns and measures of growth, adiposity, and cardiometabolic health during childhood.

The intestinal microbiota and antibiotic use have been also identified as potential modulators of early metabolic programming and development of obesity.

Considerable numbers of children and adolescents are being diagnosed with metabolic syndrome (MetS), a cluster of risk factors including abdominal fatness, hypertension, dyslipidemia, and insulin resistance, all of which increase the risk of diabetes and cardiovascular disease (CVD). One report indicates that healthy eating practices during childhood may help prevent such disturbances and reduce later CVD mortality.

Other studies assessed the effect of vitamin D supplementation on BMI and inflammatory biomarkers in obese and overweight young subjects.

The relatively new techniques of brain imaging have also been used to evaluate the brain's response to food and its association with body weight. Since the energy balance is regulated by a multifaceted system of physiological signals influencing energy intake and expenditure, any variability in the brain's response to food may be partially explained by differences in levels of metabolically active tissues throughout the body, including fat-free mass (FFM) and fat mass (FM). One study used functional magnetic resonance imaging (fMRI) to evaluate the hypothesis that the body composition of children is related to the response of the brain to food images varying in energy density (ED). Yet another study used fMRI to examine potential developmental differences in the responses of children and adults to unhealthy food (UF) cues and to determine how these responses relate to weight status.

This chapter reviews a selection of notable articles published between July 2016 and June 2017, focusing on the relation between nutrition, obesity, and MetS in childhood and young adulthood. This selection of articles published in the course of a single year indicates the range and intensity of the continuing efforts being made by researchers worldwide to confront the problem of childhood obesity.

Key articles reviewed for this chapter

Breastfeeding and Nutrition During Early Life and Risk of Childhood Obesity and Metabolic Syndrome

Predictors of infant body composition at 5 months of age: the Healthy Start Study
Sauder KA, Kaar JL, Starling AP, Ringham BM, Glueck DH, Dabelea D
J Pediatr 2017;183:94–99.e1

Targeting sleep, food, and activity in infants for obesity prevention: an RCT
Taylor BJ, Gray AR, Galland BC, Heath AM, Lawrence J, Sayers RM, Cameron S, Hanna M, Dale K, Coppell KJ, Taylor RW
Pediatrics 2017;139:pii:e20162037

Age at adiposity rebound and body mass index trajectory from early childhood to adolescence; differences by breastfeeding and maternal immigration background

Besharat Pour M, Bergström A, Bottai M, Magnusson J, Kull I, Moradi T

Pediatr Obes 2017;12:75–84

Nutrition of infants and young children (one to three years) and its effect on later health: a systematic review of current recommendations (Early Nutrition project)

Zalewski BM, Patro B, Veldhorst M, Kouwenhoven S, Crespo Escobar P, Calvo Lerma J, Koletzko B, van Goudoever JB, Szajewska H

Crit Rev Food Sci Nutr 2017;57:489–500

Intake of different types of fatty acids in infancy is not associated with growth, adiposity, or cardiometabolic health up to 6 years of age

Stroobant W, Braun KV, Kiefte-de Jong JC, Moll HA, Jaddoe VW, Brouwer IA, Franco OH, Voortman T

J Nutr 2017;147:413–420

Associations between dietary fiber intake in infancy and cardiometabolic health at school age: the Generation R study

van Gijssel RM, Braun KV, Kiefte-de Jong JC, Jaddoe VW, Franco OH, Voortman T

Nutrients 2016;8:531

Predominantly nighttime feeding and weight outcomes in infants

Cheng TS, Loy SL, Toh JY, Cheung YB, Chan JK, Godfrey KM, Gluckman PD, Saw SM, Chong YS, Lee YS, Lek N, Chong MF, Yap F

Am J Clin Nutr 2016;104:380–388

The Intestinal Microbiota and Eating Practices and their Relation to Metabolic Programming

Childhood BMI in relation to microbiota in infancy and lifetime antibiotic use

Korpela K, Zijlmans MA, Kuitunen M, Kukkonen K, Savilahti E, Salonen A, de Weerth C, de Vos WM

Microbiome 2017;5:26

Associations between school meal-induced dietary changes and metabolic syndrome markers in 8- to 11-year-old Danish children

Damsgaard CT, Ritz C, Dalskov S-T, Landberg R, Stark KD, Biltoft-Jensen A, Tetens I, Astrup A, Michaelsen KF, Lauritzen L

Eur J Nutr 2016;55:1973–1984

The Association Between Vitamin D and Inflammatory Biomarkers in Obese and Overweight Subjects

The effect of vitamin D supplementation on selected inflammatory biomarkers in obese and overweight subjects: a systematic review with meta-analysis

Jamka M, Woźniewicz M, Walkowiak J, Bogdański P, Jeszka J, Stelmach-Mardas M

Eur J Nutr 2016;55:2163–2176

Relation between milk-fat percentage, vitamin D, and BMI z score in early *childhood*
Vanderhout SM, Birken CS, Parkin PC, Lebovic G, Chen Y, O'Connor DL, Maguire JL, TARGet Kids! Collaboration

Am J Clin Nutr 2016;104:1657–1664

Vitamin D supplementation trial in infancy: body composition effects at 3 years of age in a prospective follow-up study from Montréal
Hazell TJ, Gallo S, Vanstone CA, Agellon S, Rodd C, Weiler HA

Pediatric Obesity 2017;12:38–47

Brain Imaging and Brain Response to Food

Developmental differences in the brain response to unhealthy food cues: an fMRI study of children and adults
van Meer F, van der Laan LN, Charbonnier L, Viergever MA, Adan RA, Smeets PA on behalf of the I. Family Consortium

Am J Clin Nutr 2016;104:1515–1522

Brain response to images of food varying in energy density is associated with body composition in 7- to 10-year-old children: results of an exploratory study
Fearnbach SN, English LK, Lasschuijt M, Wilson SJ, Savage JS, Fisher JO, Rolls BJ, Keller KL

Physiol Behav 2016;162:3–9

Breastfeeding and Nutrition During Early Life and Risk of Childhood Obesity and Metabolic Syndrome

Predictors of infant body composition at 5 months of age: the Healthy Start Study

Sauder KA[1], Kaar JL[1], Starling AP[2], Ringham BM[3], Glueck DH[3], Dabelea D[1, 2]

[1]Department of Pediatrics, University of Colorado School of Medicine, Aurora, CO, USA; [2]Department of Epidemiology, Colorado School of Public Health, Aurora, CO, USA; [3]Department of Biostatistics and Informatics, Colorado School of Public Health, Aurora, CO, USA

J Pediatr 2017;183:94–99.e1

Background: Intrauterine exposure to maternal obesity is associated with increased obesity in offspring across the lifespan. Greater maternal pre-pregnant BMI and gestational weight gain are both associated with greater offspring body size and adiposity at birth. However, the degree to which these associations persist into the postnatal period has not been properly investigated.

The main purpose of this analysis was to evaluate whether maternal pre-pregnant BMI, gestational weight gain, and breastfeeding exclusivity are associated independently with offspring body size and composition at 5 months of age. In addition, the analysis also aimed to determine whether these effects are independent of body composition at birth and early infant growth.

Methods: Women from obstetric clinics were recruited in early pregnancy. Data of 640 mother/ offspring pairs from early pregnancy through approximately 5 months of age were collected. Offspring body composition was assessed with air displacement plethysmography at birth and approximately at 5 months of age. Linear regression analyses examined associations between predictors and FFM, FM, and percent FM (adiposity) at approximately 5 months. Secondary models were further adjusted for body composition at birth and rapid infant growth.

Results: Greater pre-pregnant BMI and gestational weight gain were associated with greater FFM at approximately 5 months of age, but not after adjustment for FFM at birth. Greater gestational weight gain was also associated with greater FM at approximately 5 months of age, independent of FM at birth and rapid infant growth, although this did not translate to increased adiposity. Greater percent time of exclusive breastfeeding was associated with lower FFM (-311 g; $p < 0.001$), greater FM ($+224$ g; $p < 0.001$), and greater adiposity ($+3.51\%$; $p < 0.001$). Compared with offspring of non-Hispanic white mothers, offspring of Hispanic mothers had greater adiposity ($+2.72\%$; $p < 0.001$) and offspring of non-Hispanic black mothers had lower adiposity (-1.93%; $p < 0.001$). Greater adiposity at birth suggested greater adiposity at approximately 5 months of age, independent of infant feeding and rapid infant growth.

Conclusions: There are clear differences in infant body composition by demographic, perinatal, and infant feeding characteristics, although data also show that increased adiposity at birth persists through approximately 5 months of age. These findings warrant further research into implications of differences in infant body composition.

Comments   Body composition in early life influences the development of obesity during childhood and adolescence. Therefore, it is important to adequately determine body composition during the first months of life. In a similar study in 203 healthy term infants, longitudinal body composition was also investigated. Changes in body fat % occurred mainly in the first 3 months of life, supporting the concept of a critical window for adiposity development in the first 3 months of life [3].

Appetite-regulating hormones play a role in the regulation of food intake and might thus influence body composition. In 197 healthy term infants, leptin, ghrelin, and insulin were associated with FM percentage or its changes during the first 6 months of life. Formula-fed infants had a different profile of appetite-regulating hormones than breastfed infants, suggesting that lower levels of ghrelin, leptin, and insulin in breastfed infants contribute to the protective role of breastfeeding against obesity development [4]. Higher cord blood leptin was also associated with slower weight gain during infancy, and this association was driven by lower increases in adiposity, at least in early infancy [5].

Targeting sleep, food, and activity in infants for obesity prevention: an RCT

Taylor BJ[1], Gray AR[2], Galland BC[3], Heath AM[4], Lawrence J[3], Sayers RM[3], Cameron S[3], Hanna M[3], Dale K[3], Coppell KJ[5], Taylor RW[5]

Departments of [1]the Dean, Dunedin School of Medicine, [2]Preventive and Social Medicine, [3]Women's and Children's Health, [4]Human Nutrition, and [5]Medicine, University of Otago, Dunedin, New Zealand

Pediatrics 2017;139:pii:e20162037

Background: Obesity prevention studies, implemented in early life, concentrated on changing nutrition and activity in infants, with relatively little success. Although sleep is strongly associated with weight in observational research, few interventions have investigated the effectiveness of sleep modification for obesity prevention.

The aim of the study was to determine whether a conventional approach (food, activity, and breast-feeding (FAB) intervention), and/or an indirect approach (sleep intervention), to obesity prevention would result in lower BMI at 2 years of age compared with standard care.

Methods: This community-based, 2-year randomized controlled trial (RCT), allocated 802 pregnant women (≥16 years, <34 weeks' gestation) to 4 arms: control (usual care), FAB, sleep, and their combination (FAB and sleep). All groups received standard child care. FAB participants received additional support (8 contacts) promoting breastfeeding, healthy eating, and physical activity (antenatal-18 months). Sleep participants received 2 sessions (antenatal, 3 weeks) targeting prevention of sleep problems, as well as a sleep treatment program if requested (6–24 months). Combination participants received both interventions (9 contacts). BMI was measured at 24 months by researchers blinded to group allocation, and secondary outcomes (diet, physical activity, sleep) were assessed by using a questionnaire or accelerometery at multiple time points.

Results: At 2 years, 686 women remained in the study (86%). No significant intervention effect was observed for BMI at 24 months ($p = 0.086$), but there was an overall group effect for the prevalence of obesity ($p = 0.027$). Exploratory analyses found a protective effect for obesity among those receiving "sleep intervention" (sleep and combination compared with FAB and control: OR 0.54 [95% CI 0.35–0.82]). No effect was observed for "FAB intervention" (FAB and combination compared with sleep and control: OR 1.20 [95% CI 0.80–1.81]).

Conclusions: A well-developed food and activity intervention did not seem to affect children's weight status. However, further research on more intensive or longer running sleep interventions is warranted.

Comments Short sleep duration has been found to be associated with overweight and obesity in childhood. In 7,867 children aged 2–9 years, a dose-dependent inverse association between sleep duration and overweight was observed; after adjustment by geographical location, the association remained significant for sleeping less than 9 h per night (OR 2.22; 99% CI 1.64–3.02) [6]. The IDEFICS intervention was based on the intervention mapping approach identifying 6 target behaviors, including ensuring adequate sleep duration. Nocturnal sleep duration of 11/10 h or more in pre-school/school children was achieved by 37.9% of the studied sample [7]. The sleep component of the intervention did not lead to clinically relevant changes in sleep duration [8]; however, adherence to physical activity, TV, and sleep recommendations was the main driver reducing the chance of being overweight during the 2 years follow-up [9]. Behavioral interventions targeting mothers and young children as the one presented in the current study, can be delivered inexpensively and not requiring specialized training. They could help prevent the development of obesity in infants and children; however, more research is needed, with focus on sleep determinants such as sleep knowledge, practices, and related environment.

Shalitin · Moreno

Age at adiposity rebound and body mass index trajectory from early childhood to adolescence; differences by breastfeeding and maternal immigration background

Besharat Pour M[1], Bergström A[1], Bottai M[2], Magnusson J[1], Kull I[1, 3, 4], Moradi T[1, 5]

[1]Institute of Environmental Medicine, Division of Epidemiology, Karolinska Institutet, Stockholm, Sweden; [2]Institute of Environmental Medicine, Unit of Biostatistics, Karolinska Institutet, Stockholm, Sweden; [3]Department of Clinical Science and Education, Stockholm South General Hospital, Karolinska Institutet, Stockholm, Sweden; [4]Sachs' Children and Youth Hospital, Stockholm South General Hospital, Stockholm, Sweden; [5]Centre for Epidemiology and Community Medicine, Stockholm County Council, Stockholm, Sweden

Pediatr Obes 2017;12:75–84

Background: Overweight children follow a higher BMI trajectory compared to their normal weight peers. During infancy, BMI rapidly increases after birth and peaks at 12 months of age, then gradually decreases until 6 years; literature has found that BMI nadir typically occurs within the range of 3–8 years of age. Thereafter, BMI starts a second phase of increase that will continue towards adulthood BMI.

This paper aims to assess associations between breastfeeding and maternal immigration background and BMI development trajectories from age 2 to 16 years.

Methods: A cohort of children born in Stockholm during 1994 to 1996 was followed from age 2 to 16 years, with repeated measurements of height and weight at a maximum of 8-time points. The final study population included 2,278 children with complete information on breastfeeding, maternal country of birth, and BMI at least in 2-time points from 2 to 16 years of age. Age 2 years as start of follow-up was chosen to ensure temporal relationship between exposure and outcome.

Children were categorized by breastfeeding status during the first 6 months of life into 3 groups of never/short (exclusive breastfeeding <2 weeks), partial (exclusive breastfeeding 2 weeks to <6 months), and exclusively breastfeeding (exclusive breastfeeding ≥6 months). Based on maternal country of birth, children were divided into 2 groups – offspring of Swedish mothers and of foreign born mothers (immigrant mothers). Foreign born mothers were from 61 countries. BMI trajectories and age at adiposity rebound were estimated using mixed-effects linear models.

Results: BMI trajectories were different by breastfeeding and maternal immigration status (*p* value <0.0001). Compared with exclusively breastfed counterparts, never/short breastfed children of Swedish mothers had a higher BMI trajectory, whereas never/short breastfed children of immigrant mothers followed a lower BMI trajectory. The estimated age at adiposity rebound ranged from 48 to 59 months. Ages at adiposity rebound were earlier for higher BMI trajectories regardless of maternal immigration background.

Conclusions: Differences in BMI trajectories and age at adiposity rebound between offspring of immigrant and of Swedish mothers suggest a lack of beneficial association between breastfeeding and long-term BMI development among children of immigrant mothers. Given the relation between long-term BMI development and risk of overweight/obesity, these differences challenge the notion that exclusive breastfeeding is always beneficial for children's BMI development and subsequent risk of overweight/obesity.

Comments   Early adiposity rebound, when BMI rises after reaching a nadir, has been suggested as a predictor of later obesity. Therefore, adiposity rebound is considered as a suitable time period for childhood obesity prevention.

Breastfeeding for longer than 4 months seems to be a protective behavior against later obesity development. In a retrospective cohort study that included 1,812 children born in 2004, with follow-up until they were 8 years of age, breastfeeding during the first 6 months of life was not associated with a delay in the age of the adiposity rebound [10]. Concerning population differences in adiposity rebound, there is little information on this issue. There is also little information on whether childhood physical development in other populations differs from western populations. For instance, obese Japanese children developed adiposity rebound earlier than non-obese Japanese children, similar to those in Western countries reported in the literature [11].

In any case, these results highlight the importance of monitoring childhood growth so as to help identify children with early adiposity rebound who would be at risk of developing obesity later in life.

Nutrition of infants and young children (one to three years) and its effect on later health: a systematic review of current recommendations (Early Nutrition project)

Zalewski BM[1], Patro B[1], Veldhorst M[2], Kouwenhoven S[2], Crespo Escobar P[3], Calvo Lerma J[3], Koletzko B[4], van Goudoever JB[2, 5], Szajewska H[1]

[1]Department of Pediatrics, The Medical University of Warsaw, Warsaw, Poland; [2]Department of Pediatrics, VU University Medical Center Amsterdam, Amsterdam, The Netherlands; [3]Department of Pediatric Gastroenterology, La Fe University Hospital, Valencia, Spain; [4]Division of Metabolic and Nutritional Medicine, Dr. von Hauner Children's Hospital, University of Munich Medical Centre, Klinikum d. Univ. München, München, Germany; [5]Department of Pediatrics, Emma Children's Hospital, Amsterdam Medical Center, Amsterdam, The Netherlands

Crit Rev Food Sci Nutr 2017;57:489–500

Background: Evidence suggesting that nutrition early in life has consequences even in adulthood has emerged in recent decades. Nutrition-related chronic diseases, such as CVDs, obesity, type 2 diabetes, osteoporosis or some forms of cancer, have been linked to maternal and early infant nutrition. Nutrition in early life may influence metabolic programming and therefore the development of diseases later in life.

The aim of this article is to summarize, by performing a systematic review, current standards, recommendations, guidelines, and regulations (hereafter, referred to as documents) on the nutrition of children up to 3 years of age. The authors place a special emphasis on available studies on long-term effects of early nutrition, such as the risk of CVDs, hypertension, overweight, obesity, MetS, diabetes, or glucose intolerance.

Methods: MEDLINE, selected databases, and websites were searched for documents published between 2008 and January 2013. Only English language documents developed by and recognized by international and national societies and organizations were included. Position papers, scientific reports, and commentaries were also considered for inclusion.

Results: Almost 2,500 records were screened. A total of 156 publications that required further full text evaluation were identified. Forty-two documents met the inclusion criteria.

The strongest and most consistent evidence for a protective, long-term effect was documented for breastfeeding. There is a consistency across the guidelines that exclusive breastfeeding for around 6 months is a desirable goal. Partial breastfeeding as well as breastfeeding for shorter periods of time are also valuable. In general, complementary food should be introduced into the infant diet within the range of 4 to 6 months of age.

Also, limiting the intake of sodium and rapidly absorbed carbohydrates, use of a specific meal pattern, reducing the consumption of saturated fatty acids (SFAs) by replacing them with polyunsaturated fatty acids (PUFAs), and lowering the intake of trans-fatty acids, seems beneficial. Many documents did not evaluate long-term outcomes of interest, or reported insufficient or imprecise data. Inconsistency in recommendations for some outcomes and research gaps were identified.

Conclusions: The reported findings may serve as a helpful tool in planning further research, preventive actions against important diet-related diseases, and guidelines improvement.

Comments There are many aspects related with nutrition in early life that could influence the development of some conditions during childhood or even in adulthood [12]. The body of evidence is still limited but it sufficient in some areas. In most of the cases, there are recommendations with scarce scientific support. For a health professional interested in the topic, it is difficult to have a clear idea of the situation. For this reason, the current paper is important, as it compiles the available recommendations and their scientific background.

As stated in the abstract, the strongest and most consistent evidence for a protective, long-term effect of early nutrition was documented for breastfeeding. In the identified documents, several of them did not assess long-term outcomes or included insufficient data to justify the conclusions and the quality of evidence used to prepare the guidelines was not assessed. Some discrepancies in recommendations were also identified.

Another important value of this systematic review is the identification of research gaps in the literature that should support the development of further research projects. It was identified that current evidence on the long-term effects of early nutrition is based mainly on associations and not causality. Therefore, well designed and properly conducted RCTs, using strong clinical outcome measures and with relevant inclusion/exclusion criteria and adequate sample sizes should be used in the future.

Intake of different types of fatty acids in infancy is not associated with growth, adiposity, or cardiometabolic health up to 6 years of age

Stroobant W[1], Braun KV[1], Kiefte-de Jong JC[1, 2], Moll HA[3], Jaddoe VW[1, 3], Brouwer IA[4], Franco OH[1], Voortman T[5]

[1]Departments of Epidemiology and [2]Pediatrics, Erasmus Medical Center, University Medical Center, Rotterdam, The Netherlands; [3]Leiden University College, The Hague, The Netherlands; [4]Department of Health Sciences, Vrije Universiteit, Amsterdam, The Netherlands

J Nutr 2017;147:413–420

Background: The development of cardiometabolic risk factors begins early in life. Studies in adults indicate that a lower saturated and higher unsaturated fat intake is associated with a lower risk of MetS and CVDs. However, studies on fat intake in relation to cardiometabolic health during childhood are scarce.

The objective of this study was to examine the association between the intake of different types of fatty acids in early childhood and body composition and cardiometabolic health at 6 years of age in a prospective cohort study.

Methods: This study was conducted in 2,927 children participating in the Generation R study, a multiethnic, prospective, population-based cohort from fetal life onward in Rotterdam, The Netherlands. To determine their child's dietary intake, mothers completed a semi-quantitative food frequency questionnaire. Food intake was assessed when the children had a median age of 12.9 months (95%, range 12.2–18.9 months). Children's total fat intake and intakes of SFAs, monounsaturated fatty acids (MUFAs), and PUFAs were estimated as percentage of total energy intake. Children's height and weight up to age 6 years were repeatedly measured. At 6 years of age, body fat percentage with a DXA scanner, diastolic and systolic blood pressure, and serum insulin, triacylglycerol, and high density lipoprotein (HDL)-cholesterol were measured. These outcomes were combined into a cardiometabolic risk factor score. Associations of FA intake with repeated measures of height, weight, and BMI by using linear mixed models and with cardiometabolic outcomes by using linear regression models, adjusting for sociodemographic and lifestyle factors and taking into account macronutrient substitution effects were examined.

Results: In multivariable models, no associations of a higher intake of total fat or SFAs, MUFAs, or PUFAs with growth, adiposity, or cardiometabolic health when fat was consumed at the expense of carbohydrates were observed. In subsequent models, there were also no associations observed for higher MUFA or PUFA intakes at the expense of SFAs with any of the outcomes. Results did not differ by sex, ethnicity, age, or birth weight.

Conclusion: The results of this study did not support the hypothesis that intake of different types of FAs are associated with adiposity or cardiometabolic health among children.

Comments   In the adult literature, there is controversy about the effect of different macronutrients intake on obesity and other cardiovascular risk factors. This is even more so in children and adolescents, as there is scarce information in that respect. Recently, the focus is mainly on protein and free sugars intake [13]; however, there are some previous studies showing the potential effect of dietary fat intake in the development of obesity. In the STRIP study, 1,062 children were randomly assigned to an intervention group receiving biannual fat-oriented dietary counseling or to a control group at 7 months of age. The children who were overweight at 13 years of age gained more weight than their normal-weight peers by the age of 2 or 3 years onward, and girls became overweight by the age of 5 years, whereas boys only after 8 years of age; however, the intervention had no effect on the examined growth parameters [14]. In the same study, the decrease in total and saturated fat intakes in the intervention group had a positive effect on the insulin resistance index in children aged 9 years [15]. Overall, there is no consistent information on the role of total fat intake or either different fatty acids intake in relation to obesity or related cardiometabolic complications in children and adolescents. Future studies should be performed using robust methods to assess the dietary intake or biomarkers of their intake alone or a combination of both.

Associations between dietary fiber intake in infancy and cardiometabolic health at school age: the Generation R study

van Gijssel RM[1, 2], Braun KV[3], Kiefte-de Jong JC[4, 5], Jaddoe VW[6–8], Franco OH[9], Voortman T[10]

[1]The Department of Epidemiology, Erasmus MC, University Medical Center, Rotterdam, The Netherlands; [2]The Generation R Study Group, Erasmus MC, University Medical Center, Rotterdam The Netherlands; [3]Department of Global Public Health, Leiden University, The Hague, The Netherlands; [4]The Department of Pediatrics, Erasmus MC, University Medical Center, Rotterdam, The Netherlands

Nutrients 2016;8:531

Background: In adults, dietary fiber intake is beneficial for various aspects of cardiometabolic health, such as lower insulin and cholesterol concentrations and lower blood pressure. However, whether this already occurs in early childhood is unclear.

Aim: The aim was to assess if there are associations between dietary fiber intake in infancy and cardiometabolic health in children.

Methods: Population-based cohort in Rotterdam, The Netherlands. Information on dietary fiber intake at a median age of 12.9 months was collected using a food-frequency questionnaire in 2,032 children. The population for analysis ranged from 1,314 to 1,995 children, per cardiometabolic outcome. The total dietary fiber intake was calculated using the Dutch Food Composition database (NEVO, Netherlands Voedingsstoffenbestand), where dietary fiber is defined as plant cell wall components that are not digestible by human digestive enzymes. Dietary fiber was adjusted for energy intake using the residual method. At a median age of 5.9 years, children visited the hospital, where they were examined. As a primary outcome, cardiometabolic risk factors including body fat percentage, high-density lipoprotein cholesterol, insulin and triglyceride concentrations, and diastolic and systolic blood pressure were used. These variables were expressed in age- and sex-specific standard deviation scores, and the total score was computed.

Results: In models adjusted for several parental and child covariates, a higher dietary fiber intake was associated with a lower cardiometabolic risk factor score. Cardiometabolic factors were observed individually, 1 g/day higher energy-adjusted dietary fiber intake was associated with 0.026 SDS higher HDL-cholesterol (95% CI 0.009–0.042), and 0.020 SDS lower triglycerides (95% CI –0.037 to –0.003), but not with body fat, insulin, or blood pressure. Results were similar for dietary fiber with and without adjustment for energy intake.

Conclusions: The observed findings suggest that higher dietary fiber intake in infancy may be associated with better cardiometabolic health in later childhood.

Comments   Another player when assessing the potential role of nutrients in the development of obesity and related cardiometabolic disorders during childhood is dietary fiber. However, there is also scarce information in this regard, just coming from cross-sectional studies. In a cross-sectional study in Danish children aged 8–11, dietary whole-grain and fiber intakes were not associated with the FM index but were inversely associated with serum insulin concentrations [16]. In adolescents, energy-adjusted water-soluble fiber and water insoluble fiber were positively associated with body fat percentage, waist to height ratio, and low-density lipoprotein cholesterol, while energy-adjusted water-soluble fiber was inversely associated with serum fasting glucose [17]. Further studies, especially well designed clinical trials are necessary to confirm the beneficial effects of total dietary fiber and its different types in terms of obesity development and related metabolic conditions in children and adolescents.

Predominantly nighttime feeding and weight outcomes in infants

Cheng TS[1], Loy SL[3, 5], Toh JY[7], Cheung YB[4, 8], Chan JK[2, 3, 5], Godfrey KM[9, 10], Gluckman PD[7, 11], Saw SM[12], Chong YS[7, 13], Lee YS[7, 14], Lek N[1, 5], Chong MF[6, 14], Yap F[1, 5, 15]

Departments of [1]Pediatrics and [2]Reproductive Medicine and [3]KK Research Center, KK Women's and Children's Hospital, Singapore; [4]Center for Quantitative Medicine, [5]Duke-NUS Medical School, Singapore; [6]Clinical Nutrition Research Center, [7]Singapore Institute for Clinical Sciences, Agency for Science, Technology and Research, Singapore; [8]Tampere Center for Child Health Research, University of Tampere and Tampere University Hospital, Tampere, Finland; [9]Medical Research Council Lifecourse Epidemiology Unit, University of Southampton, Southampton, UK; [10]National Institute for Health Research Southampton Biomedical Research Center, University of Southampton and University Hospital Southampton National Health Service Foundation Trust, Southampton, UK; [11]Liggins Institute, University of Auckland, Auckland, New Zealand; [12]Saw Swee Hock School of Public Health and Departments of [13]Obstetrics and Gynaecology and [14]Pediatrics, Yong Loo Lin School of Medicine, National University of Singapore, Singapore; [15]Lee Kong Chian School of Medicine, Nanyang Technological University, Singapore

Am J Clin Nutr 2016;104:380–388

This manuscript is also discussed in Chapter 6, pages 111–128.

Background: The influence of circadian feeding patterns on weight outcomes has been shown in animal and human studies but not in very young children. Adults who consumed greater energy in the evening tend to be overweight or obese.

The study aimed to assess the association between infant's circadian feeding patterns at 12 months of age and the subsequent growth and weight status after 1 year.

Methods: Mothers from the ongoing prospective mother-offspring cohort study GUSTO (Growing Up in Singapore Towards Healthy Outcomes) in Singapore were included. A total of 349 mothers answered a 24-h dietary recall administered by trained clinical staff with the use of a 5-stage, multiple-pass interviewing technique to record food intakes and feeding times of the mothers' children on the previous day, when the infants had 12 months of age. Mothers were also asked whether the assessed infant food intakes were typical or atypical compared with those on other unrecorded days. Predominantly daytime (07.00–18.59; $n = 282$) and predominantly nighttime (19.00–06.59; $n = 67$) feeding infants were defined by whether daytime energy intake was >50% or <50% of total energy intake. BMI-for-age z scores were computed using the World Health Organization (WHO) Child Growth Standards 2006 to determine changes in BMI-for-age z scores from 12 to 24 months of age and weight status at 24 months of age. Multivariable linear and logistic regression analyses were performed.

Results: Compared with predominantly daytime feeding, predominantly nighttime feeding was associated with a higher BMI-for-age z scores gain from 12 to 24 months of age (adjusted $\beta = 0.38$; 95% CI 0.11–0.65; $p = 0.006$) and increased risk of becoming overweight at 24 months of age (adjusted OR 2.78; 95% CI 1.11–6.97; $p = 0.029$) with adjustments for maternal age, education, ethnicity, monthly household income, parity, infant BMI-for-age z scores at 12 months of age, feeding mode in the first 6 months of life, and total daily energy intake.

Conclusions: The study suggests that the role of daily distribution of energy consumption in weight regulation begins in infancy. The feeding of infants predominantly during nighttime hours was associated with adiposity gain and risk of overweight in early childhood. The inclusion of advice on the appropriate feeding time may be considered when implementing strategies to prevent childhood obesity.

Comments   Food consumption timing is a new issue in infant nutrition. In adults, unusual feeding time may produce a disruption of the circadian system with further unhealthy consequences. Taking into account that feeding is the source of energy for adipose tissue, the time of feeding, particularly for high-energy content meals seems to be a relevant question for the development of obesity from childhood. These findings may be justified by the presence of an active circadian clock in different organs related to food intake; this is the case for stomach, intestine, pancreas or liver [18].

In a study in pregnant women, predominantly nighttime feeding was associated with higher fasting glucose concentrations in lean but not in overweight women; this finding suggests that the effect of timing of maternal feeding on glucose homeostasis may be dependent of adiposity [19]. Also, in a prospective birth cohort study assessing dietary intakes of 12-months-old infants and their respective feeding times using a 24-hours dietary recall, the timing of feeding at 12 months was associated with daily energy and macronutrient intakes, and feeding mode during early infancy [20]. No other study assessed the relationship between timing of infant feeding and later obesity development.

Despite the very scarce literature on the issue in infants, children or adolescents, it seems there are different patterns of energy intake during the day and they could influence later obesity development and metabolism.

The Intestinal Microbiota and Eating Practices and their Relation to Metabolic Programming

Childhood BMI in relation to microbiota in infancy and lifetime antibiotic use

Korpela K[1], Zijlmans MA[2], Kuitunen M[3], Kukkonen K[4], Savilahti E[3], Salonen A[1], de Weerth C[2], de Vos WM[1, 5]

[1]Immunobiology Research Program, Department of Bacteriology and Immunology, University of Helsinki, Helsinki, Finland; [2]Department of Developmental Psychology, Behavioural Science Institute, Radboud University Nijmegen, Nijmegen, The Netherlands; [3]Children's Hospital, University of Helsinki and Helsinki University Central Hospital, Helsinki, Finland; [4]Skin and Allergy Hospital, Department of Paediatrics, Helsinki University Central Hospital, Helsinki, Finland; [5]Laboratory of Microbiology, Wageningen University, Wageningen, The Netherlands

Microbiome 2017;5:26

Background: The intestinal microbiota and use of antibiotic have been identified as potential modulators of early metabolic programming and weight development.

The aim was to assess if the early microbiota composition is associated with later BMI, and if the use of antibiotic modifies this association.

Methods: The fecal microbiota composition at 3 months and the BMI (calculated by measurements of weight and height) at 5–6 years were analyzed in 2 cohorts of healthy children born vaginally at term in The Netherlands ($n = 87$) and Finland ($n = 75$). Records of lifetime antibiotic use were obtained.

Results: The microbiota compositions differed clearly between the countries. The background variables: country, birth weight, breastfeeding duration, and total lifetime antibiotic use explained 11% of the BMI variation. The only significant contributor to BMI was birth weight ($p < 0.001$). Antibiotic use had a nearly significant positive association with BMI ($p = 0.06$). Children with a low relative abundance of Actinobacteria and a high relative abundance of Firmicutes at the age of 3 months were likely to attain a higher BMI at the age of 5–6 years, but only if they received several courses of antibiotics.

Conclusions: The intestinal microbiota of infants is predictive of later BMI and may serve as an early indicator of obesity risk. The influence on BMI appears to depend on later antibiotic use.

Comments   The human gut microbiota consists of up to 100 trillion microbes that exist in largely symbiotic relationship with their human hosts, and carry at least 150 times more genes than are present in the entire human genome [21, 22]. There is significant cross-sectional variability in the microbiota between individuals and longitudinal variability within individuals. Both the abundance and the composition of the gut microbial population are influenced by genetic and environmental factors such as diet, medication, weight, and overall metabolic state of the host. In turn, and based on animal studies, the microbiota is capable of secreting or altering the production of molecules that affect both energy balance (weight gain/loss) and energy stores (FM) [23, 24].

The establishment of the gut microbial population in the neonate is a complex process that may involve interactions between the maternal and fetal genes and environment. These interactions may begin before birth and progress through multiple stages under the influence of various internal factors, such as the early decline in the abundance of oxygen in the gut that influences the balance of aerobes and anaerobes, and external factors such as diet [25]. Vaginally delivered neonates have larger populations of *Bacteroides* and *Bifidobacteria* species than those born by C-section [26] that have been reported to persist for months to years [25]. The observations that increased Bacteroidetes populations are present in both obese children and children born by C-section [27] suggest that the infant microbiome may contribute to the subsequent increased risk of obesity in children [28] and young adults [29] delivered by C-section. Similarly, maternal exposure to antibiotics in late pregnancy or exposure in early infancy are associated with decreased bacterial diversity of the first stool of the neonate, reduced abundance of lactobacilli and bifidobacteria in the infant gut, and an approximately 80% increased risk of childhood obesity [30].

The current study demonstrated that the intestinal microbiota of infants is predictive of later BMI and may serve as an early indicator of obesity risk, but only if these infants received several courses of antibiotics.

Identification of factors that increase the risk of excessive weight gain can help promote preventive strategies. The microbiota may represent a biomarker for assessing individual risks of excessive weight gain, and is a likely candidate for metabolic programming of infants. Moreover, the aggressive hands-on approach of prescribing antibiotics in early life has to also consider the long-term outcome of the risk of becoming obese.

Shalitin · Moreno

Associations between school meal-induced dietary changes and metabolic syndrome markers in 8- to 11-year-old Danish children

Damsgaard CT[1], Ritz C[1], Dalskov S-T[1], Landberg R[2, 3], Stark KD[4], Biltoft-Jensen A[5], Tetens I[5], Astrup A[1], Michaelsen KF[1], Lauritzen L[1]

[1]Department of Nutrition, Exercise and Sports, Faculty of Science, University of Copenhagen, Frederiksberg, Denmark; [2]Department of Food Science, Swedish University of Agricultural Sciences, Uppsala, Sweden; [3]Nutritional Epidemiology Unit, Institute for Environmental Medicine, Karolinska Institutet, Stockholm, Sweden; [4]Department of Kinesiology, University of Waterloo, Waterloo, ON, Canada; [5]Division of Nutrition, National Food Institute, Technical University of Denmark, Søborg, Denmark

Eur J Nutr 2016;55:1973–1984

Background: Consumption of meals rich in fish, vegetables, and potatoes with reduced intakes of fat can improve the blood pressure, homeostatic model assessment insulin resistance (HOMA-IR), and plasma triacylglycerol.

The aim of the present study was to evaluate whether intake of key dietary components of Nordic school meals are associated with MetS markers during 6-month intervention.

Methods: Data from 7-day dietary records and measurements of blood pressure, waist circumference, android/total FM assessed by dual-energy X-ray absorptiometry, whole-blood docosahexaenoic acid (DHA, 22:6n-3), an indicator of fish intake, and fasting blood MetS markers were collected at baseline, 3 and 6 months from children ($n = 523$). These parameters were analyzed in linear mixed-effects models adjusted for puberty, growth, and fasting.

Results: Whole-blood DHA was negatively associated with HOMA-IR ($p < 0.001$) and triacylglycerol ($p < 0.0001$). Potato intake was positively associated with waist circumference ($p < 0.01$). Intakes of whole-grain, dietary fiber, protein, and fat were not associated with any of the MetS markers.

Conclusions: DHA in whole-blood was the main diet-related predictor of the beneficial effects of the school meals on MetS markers.

Comments The school food environment, including when and where children obtain food and the types of options available during the school day, plays an important role in children's consumption patterns. Thus, childhood obesity prevention efforts often focus on altering the school food environment as a mechanism for improving student dietary intake. Healthy eating practices during childhood may also help prevent metabolic disturbances and reduce later CVD mortality.

Children from most Western populations have low consumption of fish and coarse vegetables and thereby eat few dietary fibers and too much sugar and saturated fat, relative to dietary guidelines. Nordic diets rich in fish, fruits, berries, vegetables, whole-grains, and nuts have been shown to improve CVD risk factors and have been associated with reduced mortality in adults [31]. Increased intake of n-3 long-chain polyunsaturated fatty acids and reduced intake of saturated fat can improve the blood pressure, insulin sensitivity, and lipid profile [32], and vegetable intake has been associated with reduced risk of MetS in adults.

Danish children get 40–45% of their daily energy intake in school and in after-school centers that offer the opportunity to test the impact of healthy diets on cardiometabolic health in children. This study found that insulin resistance and plasma triacylglycerol were inversely associated with whole-blood DHA. Surprisingly, neither intakes of whole-grain, dietary fiber, protein or fat were associated with the MetS markers.

Therefore, fish and n-3 long-chain polyunsaturated fatty acids are key components in a healthy diet with potential for prevention of MetS from childhood.

One of the study limitation is that the diet assessment was based on dietary recordings, that is subject to both imprecision and inaccuracy, including selective under- and over-reporting, especially in children. Another limitation is the generalization of the study results, since in many countries fish consumption by children is much lower than in the Danish population.

However, it suggests that school can offer a good opportunity of nutritional intervention to improve the metabolic outcome by healthier food consumption.

The Association Between Vitamin D and Inflammatory Biomarkers in Obese and Overweight Subjects

The effect of vitamin D supplementation on selected inflammatory biomarkers in obese and overweight subjects: a systematic review with meta-analysis

Jamka M[1], Woźniewicz M[1], Walkowiak J[2], Bogdański P[3], Jeszka J[1], Stelmach-Mardas M[2, 4]

[1]Department of Human Nutrition and Hygiene, Poznan University of Life Sciences, Poznan, Poland; [2]Department of Paediatric Gastroenterology and Metabolic Diseases, Poznan University of Medical Sciences, Poznan, Poland; [3]Department of Education and Obesity Treatment and Metabolic Disorders, Poznan University of Medical Sciences, Poznan, Poland; [4]Department of Epidemiology, German Institute of Human Nutrition, Potsdam-Rehbrücke, Nuthetal, Germany

Eur J Nutr 2016;55:2163–2176

Background: Obesity is strongly associated with a low-grade chronic inflammation. There is an inverse association between vitamin D level and total body fat and visceral obesity. Vitamin D can also play a role in immune activation and inflammation.

The aim of the current review was to assess the effect of vitamin D supplementation on selected inflammatory biomarkers in obese and overweight subjects.

Methods: The search process was based on the selection of publications of RCTs in the databases of: PubMed, Web of knowledge, Scopus, the Cochrane Library, and Embase. The study quality was assessed by a 9-point scoring with high-quality study defined by a threshold of ≥7 points. Thirteen RCTs, consisting of 1,955 overweight and obese subjects (mean age range 13.6–71.7 years), were included. Changes in the concentration of 25-hydroxyvitamin D (25[OH]D), C-reactive protein, tumor necrosis factor-α, and interleukin-6 were assessed.

Results: The baseline levels of 25OHD suggested common vitamin D deficiency or insufficiency in the analyzed population. Vitamin D supplementation increased the plasma concentrations of 25OHD in each of the intervention groups achieving the mean levels of 20.1–80.0 ng/mL. The findings of this meta-analysis did not show statistically significant impact of vitamin D supplementation on selected pro-inflammatory cytokines (tumor necrosis factor-α and interleukin-6) and C-reactive protein.

Conclusions: The current findings suggest that vitamin D supplementation does not have a significant influence on changes in the levels of common inflammatory biomarkers in obese and overweight subjects.

Comments Vitamin D deficiency and cardiometabolic risk factors are common in obese adolescents. Observational studies demonstrate an inverse relationship among serum 25OHD and obesity, insulin resistance, and inflammatory cytokines.

Therefore, a systematic review based on RCTs to examine the association between oral vitamin D supplementation and circulating inflammatory biomarkers of overweight/obese subjects is essential. However, the current meta-analysis is limited by the small number of available studies concerning the described topic with limited number of participants. Additionally, the combined supplementation with vitamin D and calcium makes the effect difficult to distinguish between those 2 components. Furthermore, the dose of supplied vitamin D in the analyzed studies and the duration of the supplementation were different and could influence the full interpretation of the collected data. No information was available on long-term changes in cytokine levels in obese and overweight subjects that could strongly support the merit of vitamin D supplementation. Thus, RCTs with long-term follow-up should be applied for future investigations to give a better answer.

Relation between milk-fat percentage, vitamin D, and BMI z score in early childhood

Vanderhout SM[1–3], Birken CS[4–6], Parkin PC[4–6], Lebovic G[3, 6], Chen Y[3], O'Connor DL[3], Maguire JL[1–6]
TARGet Kids! Collaboration

[1]Department of Nutritional Sciences, University of Toronto, Toronto, Ontario, Canada; [2]Department of Paediatrics, and [3]Li Ka Shing Knowledge Institute, St. Michael's Hospital, Toronto, Ontario, Canada; [4]Department of Paediatrics, and [5]Division of Paediatric Medicine and the Paediatric Outcomes Research Team, The Hospital for Sick Children, Toronto, Ontario, Canada; [6]Child Health Evaluative Sciences, The Hospital for Sick Children, Peter Gilgan Centre for Research and Learning, Toronto, Ontario, Canada

Am J Clin Nutr 2016;104:1657–1664

Background: Recommendations for children older than 2 years advice reduced milk-fat consumption to reduce childhood obesity.

The objectives of the current cross-sectional study were: to explore the association between milk-fat percentage and both BMI z score (zBMI) and venous 25(OH)D, and to assess whether milk volume consumed modified this relation.

Methods: Healthy children aged 12–72 months were recruited from 9 primary health care practices within The Applied Research Group for Kids (TARGet Kids!) research group in Toronto, Canada. A linear regression analysis was used to examine the relation between milk-fat percentage and child 25(OH)D and zBMI concurrently.

Results: Among the included children ($n = 2,745$) there was a positive association between milk-fat percentage and 25(OH)D ($p = 0.006$) and a negative association with the zBMI ($p < 0.0001$). Participants who drank whole milk had a 5.4-nmol/L (95% CI 4.32–6.54) higher median 25(OH)D concentration and a 0.72 lower (95% CI 0.68–0.76) zBMI score than children who drank 1% milk. The consumed milk volume modified the effect of milk-fat percentage on 25(OH)D ($p = 0.003$) but not on zBMI ($p = 0.77$).

Conclusions: Whole milk consumption among healthy young children was associated with higher vitamin D stores and lower BMI.

Comments Fortified cow milk is a contributor of vitamin D and dietary fat in children.
Current guidelines for cow's milk consumption in children older than age 2 years suggest 1 or 2% milk to reduce the risk of obesity. Given that milk is the main dietary source of vitamin D in young children and that vitamin D is fat soluble, it was logical to hypothesize that 25(OH)D concentration may be positively associated with the fat content of milk. Since the current study demonstrated that whole milk consumption among healthy young children was associated with higher vitamin D stores, current guidelines may have the paradoxical effect of limiting 25(OH)D concentration, and consumption of milk with higher fat content may be helpful in optimizing both vitamin D stores and adiposity.

The limitations of this study include: the cross-sectional design, in which causality and its direction cannot be established between the exposure and outcomes. Data collection for milk consumption was reported by parents, which may be subject to recall bias, and 56% of the children in the study regularly consumed a vitamin D-containing supplement.

Longitudinal and intervention studies are needed to confirm the current findings and examine clinical outcomes related to both serum 25(OH)D concentrations and adiposity in children.

Vitamin D supplementation trial in infancy: body composition effects at 3 years of age in a prospective follow-up study from Montréal

Hazell TJ[1], Gallo S[2], Vanstone CA[3], Agellon S[3], Rodd C[4], Weiler HA[3]

[1]Department of Kinesiology and Physical Education, Wilfrid Laurier University, Waterloo, ON, Canada; [2]Department of Nutrition and Food Studies, George Mason University, Fairfax, VI, USA; [3]School of Dietetics and Human Nutrition, McGill University, Montréal, QC, Canada; [4]Winnipeg Children's Hospital, University of Manitoba, Winnipeg, MB, Canada

Pediatric Obesity 2017;12:38–47

Background: Circulating 25(OH)D concentrations positively associate with lean body composition in adolescents. Whether vitamin D positively relates to lean body composition in younger children is unknown. Addressing this knowledge gap could improve the understanding of the nutritional and environmental factors associated with healthy growth and body composition from birth to early childhood. The aim was to evaluate how vitamin D supplementation in infancy affects the body composition at 3 years of age.

Methods: This report is an observational follow-up of children 3 years of age that participated in a double-blind randomized trial of one-month-old healthy, breastfed infants ($n = 132$) randomly assigned to receive oral vitamin D_3 supplements of 400, 800, 1,200, or 1,600 IU/day during the first year of life. Body composition was measured using dual-energy X-ray absorptiometry and plasma 25(OH)D concentrations by liquid chromatography tandem mass spectrometry.

Results: Anthropometry, body composition, diet, activity, and demographics were similar across dosage groups at 3 years. The mean 25(OH)D concentration from 1 month to 3 years was higher ($p < 0.001$) in the 1,200 IU group than in the 800 and 400 IU groups. Children with 25(OH)D concentrations >75 nmol/L had lower FM (~450 g; $p = 0.049$). In multiple linear regression, mean 25(OH)D was associated with lean mass percent ($p = 0.042$), FM ($p = 0.048$), and body fat percentage ($p = 0.045$).

Conclusions: While there were no differences in vitamin D status or body composition at 3-year across the different vitamin D dosage groups, this study provides novel findings that suggest higher plasma 25(OH)D concentrations early in life being associated with leaner body composition.

Comments The possible mechanism for the importance of vitamin D to a leaner body composition is not fully understood. There is a large body of growing evidence showing that dairy products, calcium, and vitamin D intake play a role in the regulation of body FM [33]. Data also indicate that vitamin D may increase the lean body mass and inhibit the development of adipocytes. These effects of vitamin D may be mediated by 1,25(OH)2D3 or via suppression of PTH [34]. It has been suggested that high levels of 1α,25,dihydroxyvitamin D and iPTH can modulate intracellular Ca^{+2} concentrations, so increasing Ca^{+2} flux to adiposities, which stimulate fatty acid synthase, may increase lipogenesis and inhibit lipolysis [35].

Evidence implies that high calcium and/or vitamin D intakes can repress fatty acid synthase by decreasing intracellular Ca^{+2} in adiposities [36].

The limitation of the present study is that all children receiving at least 400 IU/day of vitamin from 1 to 12 months likely contributed to the very good vitamin D status >50 nmol/L and precluded studying children with lower vitamin D status. Overall, data of the present study suggest that children with higher vitamin D status over their first 3 years have a leaner body composition and that efforts to achieve healthy status targets should be made through ensuring adequate dietary or supplemental vitamin D intakes. However, more research is certainly warranted to establish how 25(OH)D contributes to a leaner body composition.

Brain Imaging and Brain Response to Food

Developmental differences in the brain response to unhealthy food cues: an fMRI study of children and adults

van Meer F[1,2], van der Laan LN[1,2], Charbonnier L[1,2], Viergever MA[1,2], Adan RA[2], Smeets PA[1-3] on behalf of the I. Family Consortium

[1]Image Sciences Institute and [2]University Medical Center Utrecht, Utrecht, Netherlands; [3]Division of Human Nutrition, Wageningen University and Research Centre, Wageningen, The Netherlands

Am J Clin Nutr 2016;104:1515–1522

Background: In modern societies, there is an abundance of food cues that may promote overconsumption. In light of the current rise in childhood obesity, it is crucial to investigate the neural mechanisms underlying food selection and overconsumption in children. Food selection is mainly guided by the visual system, and the sight of food leads to an array of responses ranging from preparation for food ingestion (cephalic-phase responses) to the desire to eat and hedonic evaluation. Brain areas most consistently activated by food viewing in children correspond with the appetitive brain network and largely overlap with those found in adults. However, children may not activate areas important for inhibitory control. Children may be particularly susceptible to food cues because their brain is still developing.

The aim was to examine potential developmental differences in children's and adults' responses to food cues, and to determine how these responses relate to weight status.

Methods: The study included children aged 10–12 years ($n = 27$) and adults aged 32–52 years ($n = 32$). fMRI was performed during a food-viewing task in which UF and healthy food (HF) pictures were presented.

Results: In children, there was a stronger response to UF than to HF pictures in the right temporal/occipital gyri and left precentral gyrus. Children with a higher BMI had lower activation in the bilateral dorsolateral prefrontal cortex while viewing unhealthy compared with HFs.

In adults, there was a stronger response to UF than to HF pictures in the bilateral middle occipital gyrus and the right calcarine sulcus. There were no correlations between brain activation in the UF > HF contrast and BMI.

Children had a stronger response to UFs compared with HFs than adults in the left precentral gyrus. When including healthiness ratings, liking ratings, hunger ratings, time since last meal, or Tanner stages as covariates in the fMRI analyses, the clusters found did not change. The difference between children and adults remained the same when only the parents of the included children were considered in the analysis.

Conclusions: Children activated the left precentral gyrus more than adults did in response to UF compared with HF pictures. Furthermore, children with a higher BMI had lower activation in the bilateral left dorsolateral prefrontal cortex while viewing UFs compared with HFs.

This study demonstrated that children have stronger activation than adults in brain sites implicated in motivation in response to UFs, with decreased activation in inhibitory areas in children with higher BMIs. This suggests that children who are overweight may have less control over their motivational responses toward foods.

Comments   In the field of functional neuroimaging, food stimuli, in comparison with non-food objects, activate occipital, limbic and paralimbic, and prefrontal areas. By far the most widely used technique in this research field is fMRI. This neuroimaging method measures the change in blood flow (indicated by the blood oxygen level-dependent [BOLD] signal) that is related to the neural activity in the human brain. fMRI has a number of advantages over other imaging modalities used in behavioral neuroscience: unlike nuclear techniques, it is entirely noninvasive, and its spatial resolution is much better than that achieved by magnetoencephalography and electroencephalography; furthermore, it has sufficient temporal resolution to observe patterns of neuronal activity in the entire brain in few seconds.

Functional neuroimaging studies examining brain activation in response to food images have identified brain regions related to both reward (limbic and paralimbic regions) and cognitive control (prefrontal cortices) in children [37, 38].

The finding of this study indicates that children are more susceptible to UF cues than adults, especially if they are overweight. This calls for better protection of children from targeted food marketing to prevent the overconsumption of UFs.

However, to better assess the effect of age on UF and HF cue reactivity, the results should be reproduced in a longitudinal fMRI study. Future studies should ideally take into account food intake as well to be able to clarify the link between food-cue reactivity and dietary behavior.

Brain response to images of food varying in energy density is associated with body composition in 7- to 10-year-old children: results of an exploratory study

Fearnbach SN[1], English LK[1], Lasschuijt M[2], Wilson SJ[3], Savage JS[1], Fisher JO[4], Rolls BJ[1], Keller KL[1, 5]

[1]Department of Nutritional Sciences, The Pennsylvania State University, University Park, PA, USA; [2]Division of Human Nutrition, Wageningen University, Wageningen, The Netherlands; [3]Department of Psychology, The Pennsylvania State University, University Park, PA, USA; [4]Center for Obesity Research and Education, Department of Social and Behavioral Sciences, Temple University, Philadelphia, PA, USA; [5]Department of Food Science, The Pennsylvania State University, University Park, PA, USA

Physiol Behav 2016;162:3–9

Background: Energy balance is regulated by a complex system of peripheral and central physiological signals that rise from compartments of adipose and lean tissue, as well as the gastrointestinal tract and accessory organs, to influence energy intake and expenditure. It is not known whether the effects of FM and FFM on energy balance are mediated by processes in appetite-regulating centers of the brain. Variability in the brain's response to food could partially be explained by differences in levels of metabolically active tissues (FM and FFM) throughout the body. The aim of this study was to determine the association between children's body composition, compartmentalized into FFM and FM, and brain activation in response to images of food that vary by ED, a measure of energy content per weight of food.

Methods: This was a cross-sectional study with a community-based sample of 36 children aged 7–10 years. The body composition was measured using bioelectrical impedance. Brain response to High (>1.5 kcal/g) and Low (<1.5 kcal/g) ED food images, and control images were measured by fMRI.

Multi-subject random effects general linear model and 2-factor repeated measures analysis of variance were used to test for the main effects of ED (high ED vs. low ED) in a priori defined brain regions of interest previously implicated in energy homeostasis and reward processing. Pearson's correlations were then calculated between activation in these regions for various contrasts (high ED-low ED, high ED-control, low ED-control) and child body composition (FFM index, FM index, % body fat (BF).

Results: Across the whole sample, BOLD activation was greater for high ED foods relative to low ED foods in the left thalamus ($p < 0.05$), which functions in sensory processing. BOLD activation for high ED relative to low ED foods in the right substantia nigra was positively correlated with children's FFM index ($p = 0.01$). Thus, greater amounts of lean body mass were associated with greater BOLD activation for higher ED foods in a region of the brain involved with dopamine signaling and reward. This association was unaffected after controlling for BMIz ($p < 0.05$) and for children's rated liking or wanting of high ED or low ED food images ($p < 0.05$). There was a trend in the direction of a negative association between the response to low ED foods in the right substantia nigra and both FM index and %BF.

Conclusions: The findings demonstrated a significant effect of ED on the thalamus (e.g., sensory processing) such that high ED foods elicited greater BOLD activation than low ED foods. However, there was heterogeneity in children's brain responses to food stimuli, such that not all children responded in the same direction or with the same magnitude. Overall, FFM but not FM, was positively associated with BOLD activation for high ED foods in a reward region of the brain, the substantia nigra. FFM is an appetitive driver. These results confirm that brain response to foods varying in energy content is related to measures of child body composition.

Comments Previous studies in adolescents and adults have demonstrated that FFM is the best predictor of meal size and daily energy intake [39, 40]. These effects on intake are attributed to the fact that FFM is the largest contributor to resting metabolic rate, and therefore total daily energy expenditure [41]. However, the underlying mechanism for how FFM affects appetite-regulating centers in the brain is not clear. The present results suggest that increases in FFM are associated with an increased reward response to high ED foods relative to low ED foods. Therefore, children with greater FFM have greater energy requirements, which may partly explain increased responsiveness to higher calorie foods relative to lower calorie options. However, body fat was not associated with the activation for high ED foods, which suggest that greater adiposity may be related to a reduced reward response to low ED food images. The direction of a negative association between the response to low ED foods in the right substantia nigra and both FMI and %BF suggest that as adiposity increases, children may be less responsive to healthier, low-calorie foods. It is important to evaluate this question further across a range of body weights to determine the generalizability of these findings.

The study limitations include the small sample size, the cross-sectional design in a homogenous sample of predominantly lean children that does not allow us to know whether these results are generalizable to other populations, or whether activation in these brain areas is a cause or a consequence of differences in body composition. It is possible that the relationship is bidirectional.

Future studies should determine whether these individual differences in brain activity can explain variability in actual eating behavior, and whether they are related to changes in children's weight status over time.

References

1 Ogden CL, Carroll MD, Kit BK, et al: Prevalence of obesity and trends in body mass index among US children and adolescents 1999–2010. JAMA 2012; 307:483–490.

2 Sedej K, Lusa L, Battelino T, Kotnik P: Stabilization of overweight and obesity in Slovenian adolescents and increased risk in those entering non-grammar secondary schools. Obes Facts 2016;9:241–250.

3 Breij LM, Kerkhof GF, De Lucia Rolfe E, et al: Longitudinal fat mass and visceral fat during the first 6 months after birth in healthy infants: support for a critical window for adiposity in early life. Pediatr Obes 2017;12:286–294.

4 Breij LM, Mulder MT, van Vark-van der Zee LC, Hokken-Koelega ACS: Appetite-regulating hormones in early life and relationships with type of feeding and body composition in healthy term infants. Eur J Nutr 2017;56:1725–1732.

5 Chaoimh CN, Murray DM, Kenny LC, Irvine AD, Hourihane JO, Kiely M: Cord blood leptin and gains in body weight and fat mass during infancy. Eur J Endocrinol 2016;175:403–410.

6 Hense S, Pohlabeln H, De Henauw S, et al: Sleep duration and overweight in European children: is the association modified by geographic region? Sleep 2011;34:885–890.

7 Kovács E, Siani A, Konstabel K, et al: IDEFICS Consortium: Adherence to the obesity-related lifestyle intervention targets in the IDEFICS study. Int J Obes (Lond) 2014;38(suppl 2):S144–S151.

8 Michels N, De Henauw S, Eiben G, et al: IDEFICS Consortium: Effect of the IDEFICS multilevel obesity prevention on children's sleep duration. Obes Rev 2015;16(suppl 2):68–77.

9 Kovács E, Hunsberger M, Reisch L, et al: IDEFICS Consortium: Adherence to combined lifestyle factors and their contribution to obesity in the IDEFICS study. Obes Rev 2015;16(suppl 2):138–150.

10 Estévez-González MD, Santana Del Pino A, Henríquez-Sánchez P, Peña-Quintana L, Saavedra-Santana P: Breastfeeding during the first 6 months of life, adiposity rebound and overweight/obesity at 8 years of age. Int J Obes (Lond) 2016;40:10–13.

11 Franchetti Y, Ide H: Socio-demographic and lifestyle factors for child's physical growth and adiposity rebound of Japanese children: a longitudinal study of the 21st century longitudinal survey in newborns. BMC Public Health 2014;14:334.

12 González-Muniesa P, Mártinez-González MA, Hu FB, et al: Obesity. Nat Rev Dis Primers 2017;3: 17034.

13 Moreno LA: Editorial Commentary: lifestyle and life-long lasting cardiovascular health. Trends Cardiovasc Med 2017;27:314–315.

14 Lagström H, Hakanen M, Niinikoski H, et al: Growth patterns and obesity development in overweight or normal-weight 13-year-old adolescents: the STRIP study. Pediatrics 2008;122:e876–e883.

15 Kaitosaari T, Rönnemaa T, Viikari J, et al: Low-saturated fat dietary counseling starting in infancy improves insulin sensitivity in 9-year-old healthy children: the Special Turku Coronary Risk Factor Intervention Project for Children (STRIP) study. Diabetes Care 2006;29:781–785.

16 Damsgaard CT, Biltoft-Jensen A, Tetens I, et al: Whole-grain intake, reflected by dietary records and biomarkers, is inversely associated with circulating insulin and other cardiometabolic markers in 8- to 11-year-old children. J Nutr 2017;147:816–824.

17 Lin Y, Huybrechts I, Vereecken C, et al: Dietary fiber intake and its association with indicators of adiposity and serum biomarkers in European adolescents: the HELENA study. Eur J Nutr 2015;54:771–782.

18 Garaulet M, Gómez-Abellán P: Timing of food intake and obesity: a novel association. Physiol Behav 2014;134:44–50.

19 Loy SL, Cheng TS, Colega MT, et al: Predominantly night-time feeding and maternal glycaemic levels during pregnancy. Br J Nutr 2016;115:1563–1570.

20 Wee PH, Loy SL, Toh JY, et al: Circadian feeding patterns of 12-month-old infants. Br J Nutr 2017;117: 1702–1710.

21 Hamady M, Knight R: Microbial community profiling for human microbiome projects: tools, techniques, and challenges. Genome Res 2009;19:1141–1152.

22 Ursell L, et al: The intestinal metabolome: an intersection between microbiota and host. Gastroenterology 2014;146:1470–1476.

23 Tagliabue A, Elli M: The role of gut microbiota in human obesity: recent findings and future perspectives. Nutr Metab Cardiovasc Dis 2013;23: 160–168.

24 Tehrani AB, Nezami BG, Gewirtz A, Srinivasan S: Obesity and its associated diseases: a role for microbiota? Neurogastroenterol Motil 2012;24:305–311.

25 Guaraldi F, Salvatori G: Effect of breast and formula feeding on gut microbiota shaping in newborns. Front Cell Infect Microbiol 2012;2:94.

26 Costello EK, Stagaman K, Dethlefsen L, Bohannan BJ, Relman DA: The application of ecological theory toward an understanding of the human microbiome. Science 2012;336:1255–1262.

27 Ravussin Y, Koren O, Spor A, et al: Responses of gut microbiota to diet composition and weight loss in lean and obese mice. Obesity (Silver Spring) 2012;20: 738–747.

28 Mueller NT, Whyatt R, Hoepner L, et al: Prenatal exposure to antibiotics, cesarean section and risk of childhood obesity. Int J Obes (Lond) 2015;39:665–670.

29 Blustein J, Attina T, Liu M, et al: Association of caesarean delivery with child adiposity from age 6 weeks to 15 years. Int J Obes (Lond) 2013;37:900–906.

30 Murphy R, Stewart AW, Braithwaite I, Beasley R, Hancox RJ, Mitchell EA; The ISAAC Phase Three Study Group: Antibiotic treatment during infancy and increased body mass index in body: an international cross-sectional study. Int J Obes 2014;38: 1115–1119.

31 Adamsson V, Reumark A, Fredriksson IB, et al: Effects of a healthy Nordic diet on cardiovascular risk factors in hypercholesterolaemic subjects: a randomized controlled trial (NORDIET). J Intern Med 2011; 269:150–159.

32 Miller PE, Van Elswyk M, Alexander DD: Long-chain omega-3 fatty acids eicosapentaenoic acid and docosahexaenoic acid and blood pressure: a meta-analysis of randomized controlled trials. Am J Hypertens 2014;27:885–896.

33 Rosenblum JL, Castro VM, Moore CE, Kaplan LM: Calcium and vitamin d supplementation is associated with decreased abdominal visceral adipose tissue in overweight and obese adults. Am J Clin Nutr 2012; 95(suppl 1):101–108.

34 Ward KA, Das G, Berry JL, et al: Vitamin d status and muscle function in post-menarchal adolescent girls. J Clin Endocrinol Metab 2009;9:559–563.

35 Zemel MB: Regulation of adiposity and obesity risk by dietary calcium: mechanisms and implications. J Am Coll Nutr 2002;21:146S–151S.

36 Zemel MB: Proposed role of calcium and dairy food components in weight management and metabolic health. Phys Sportsmed 2009;37:29–39.

37 Bruce AS, Holsen LM, Chambers RJ, et al: Obese children show hyperactivation to food pictures in brain networks linked to motivation, reward and cognitive control. Int J Obes 2010;34:1494–1500.

38 Killgore WD, Yurgelun-Todd DA: Developmental changes in the functional brain responses of adolescents to images of high and low-calorie foods. Dev Psychobiol 2005;47:377–397.

39 Blundell JE, Caudwell P, Gibbons C, et al: Body composition and appetite: fat-free mass (but not fat mass or BMI) is positively associated with self-determined meal size and daily energy intake in humans. Br J Nutr 2012;107:445–449.

40 Weise CM, Hohenadel MG, Krakoff J, Votruba SB: Body composition and energy expenditure predict ad-libitum food and macronutrient intake in humans. Int J Obes 2014;38:243–251.

41 Hopkins M, Finlayson G, Duarte C, et al: Modelling the associations between fat-free mass, resting metabolic rate and energy intake in the context of total energy balance. Int J Obes 2016;40:312–318.

Koletzko B, Shamir R, Turck D, Phillip M (eds): Nutrition and Growth: Yearbook 2018.
World Rev Nutr Diet. Basel, Karger, 2018, vol 117, pp 39–65 (DOI: 10.1159/000484499)

Term and Preterm Infants

Dominique Turck[1] · Johannes B. van Goudoever[2]

[1]Division of Gastroenterology, Hepatology and Nutrition, Department of Pediatrics, Lille University Jeanne de Flandre Children's Hospital and Faculty of Medicine, Lille, France; [2]Department of Pediatrics, Emma Children's Hospital-AMC and VU University Center, Amsterdam, The Netherlands

Introduction

The concept of evidence-based medicine has become essential for health care providers, as well as in the nutritional field. In 1992, David Sackett defined evidence-based medicine as "the conscientious, explicit, and judicious use of current best evidence in making decisions about the care of individual patients." As the best is needed for feeding preterm and term infants, it is of paramount importance to perform well-designed studies.

In the present chapter, we focused on 15 articles related to nutrition in preterm and term infants. We have selected 3 randomized clinical trials (RCTs) on vitamin D, iodine, and protein intake in premature babies during the first months of life. They add more information to the critical choice of the most adequate dietary intake in this population, to avoid not only deficiencies but also excessive intake that may contribute to a higher risk of metabolic disorders later in life. Two other papers on preterm infants assess controversial issues, that is, the role of post-discharge formula and the impact of the feeding schedule on time to achieve full enteral feeding.

Gross compositional similarity with the human milk of healthy women is not an adequate indicator of the safety and suitability of infant formula. Infant formulae (IF) should only contain components in certain amounts that serve a nutritional purpose or other benefit. Since dietary composition in infants has a major impact on short- and long-term child health and development, the scientific evidence to support modifications of IF beyond the established standards should be assessed by well-designed studies before evaluation by independent scientific bodies prior to the acceptance of introduction of such products on the market. We have selected 2 RCTs assessing, respectively, the safety and suitability of human milk oligosaccharides (HMOs) added to an infant formula, and the effect of a young child formula on the iron and vitamin D status of healthy young European children. The addition of long chain polyunsaturated fatty acid to infant formula is also a controversial issue in term infants. We selected a Cochrane Review on this topic that summarizes available data and asks for more research.

Despite a growing interest of the scientific community, there is limited scientific evidence on complementary feeding (CF), especially the time of introduction and the type of foods given. We selected 3 papers on CF: (1) an RCT on the appropriate time for introduction of complementary foods in infants born at less than 34 weeks of gestation; (2) a meta-analysis and systematic review on the timing of allergenic food introduction to the infant diet and risk of allergic or autoimmune disease; and (3) a position paper on CF by the ESPGHAN Committee on Nutrition (CoN).

Last but not least our review also includes an Australian study of food protein-induced enterocolitis syndrome (FPIES), guidelines on the diagnosis and management of FPIES and a position paper by ESPGHAN CoN on the prevention of vitamin K deficiency bleeding (VKDB) in newborn infants.

It has been a very fruitful year in terms of research in infant nutrition. New important and exciting data are available that will help all of us for the nutritional management of infants and young children.

Key articles reviewed for this chapter

Term Infants

Prevention of vitamin K deficiency bleeding in newborn infants: a position paper by the ESPGHAN Committee on Nutrition

Mihatsch WA, Braegger C, Bronsky J, Campoy C, Domellöf M, Fewtrell M, Mis NF, Hojsak I, Hulst J, Indrio F, Lapillonne A, Molgaard C, Embleton N, van Goudoever J, ESPGHAN Committee on Nutrition

J Pediatr Gastroenterol Nutr 2016;63:123–139

Long chain polyunsaturated fatty acid supplementation in infants born at term

Jasani B, Simmer K, Patole SK, Rao SC

Cochrane Database Syst Rev 2017;3:CD000376

Effects of infant formula with human milk oligosaccharides on growth and morbidity: a randomized multicenter trial

Puccio G, Alliet P, Cajozzo C, Janssens E, Corsello G, Sprenger N, Wernimont S, Egli D, Gosoniu L, Steenhout P

J Pediatr Gastroenterol Nutr 2017;64:624–631

First infant formula type and risk of islet autoimmunity in The Environmental Determinants of Diabetes in the Young (TEDDY) Study

Hummel S, Beyerlein A, Tamura R, Uusitalo U, Aronsson CA, Yang J, Riikonen R, Lernmark A, Rewers MJ, Hagopian WA, She JX, Simell OG, Toppari J, Ziegler AG, Akolkar B, Krischer JP, Virtanen SM, Norris JM and the TEDDY Study Group

Diabetes Care 2017;40:398–404

Food protein-induced enterocolitis syndrome in Australia: a population-based study, 2012–2014

Mehr S, Frith K, Barnes EH, Campbell DE, on behalf of the FPIES Study Group

J Allergy Clin Immunol 2017;140:1323–1330

International consensus guidelines for the diagnosis and management of food protein-induced enterocolitis syndrome: Executive Summary – Workgroup Report of the Adverse Reactions to Foods Committee, American Academy of Allergy, Asthma and Immunology

Nowak-Wegrzyn A, Chehade M, Groetch ME, Spergel JM, Wood RA, Allen KJ, Atkins D, Bahna S, Barad AV, Berin C, Brown Whitehorn T, Burks WA, Caubet JC, Cianferoni C, Conte M, Davis C, Fiocchi A, Grimshaw K, Gupta R, Hofmeister B, Hwang JB, Katz Y, Konstantinou GN, Leonard SA, Lightdale J, McGhee S, Mehr S, Miceli Sopo S, Monti G, Muraro A, Noel SK, Nomura I, Noone S, Sampson HA, Schultz F, Sicherer SH, Thompson CC, Turner PJ, Venter C, Westcott-Chavez A, Greenhawt M

J Allergy Clin Immunol 2017;139:1111–1126

Complementary feeding: a position paper by the European Society for Paediatric Gastroenterology, Hepatology, and Nutrition (ESPGHAN) Committee on Nutrition

Fewtrell M, Bronsky J, Campoy C, Domellöf M, Embleton N, Mis NF, Hojsak I, Hulst JM, Indrio F, Lapillonne A, Molgaard C

J Pediatr Gastroenterol Nutr 2017;64:119–132

Timing of allergenic food introduction to the infant diet and risk of allergic or autoimmune disease. A systematic review and meta-analysis

Ierodiakonou D, Garcia-Larsen V, Logan A, Groome A, Cunha S, Chivinge J, Robinson Z, Geoghegan N, Jarrold K, Reeves T, Tagiyeva-Milne N, Nurmatov U, Trivella M, Leonardi-Bee J, Boyle RJ

JAMA 2016;316:1181–1192

Complementary feeding at 4 versus 6 months of age for preterm infants born at less than 34 weeks of gestation: a randomised, open-label, multicentre trial

Gupta S, Agarwal R, Aggarwal KC, Chellani H, Duggal A, Arya S, Bhatia S, Sankar MJ, Sreenivas V, Jain V, Gupta AK, Deorari AK, Paul VK; Investigators of the CF trial

Lancet Glob Health 2017;5:e501–e511

A micronutrient-fortified young-child formula improves the iron and vitamin D status of healthy young European children: a randomized, double-blind controlled trial

Akkermans MD, Eussen SR, van der Horst-Graat JM, van Elburg RM, van Goudoever JB, Brus F

Am J Clin Nutr 2017;105:391–399

Preterm Infants

Randomized trial of two doses of vitamin D3 in preterm infants <32 weeks: Dose impact on achieving desired serum 25(OH)D3 in a NICU population

Anderson-Berry A, Thoene M, Wagner J, Lyden E, Jones G, Kaufmann M, Van Ormer M, Hanson C

PLoS One 2017;12:e0185950

Follow-up of a randomized trial on postdischarge nutrition in preterm-born children at age 8 years

Ruys CA, van de Lagemaat M, Finken MJ, Lafeber HN

Am J Clin Nutr 2017;106:549–558

Supplemental Iodide for preterm infants and developmental outcomes at 2 years: an RCT

Williams FLR, Ogston S, Hume R, Watson J, Stanbury K, Willatts P, Boelen A, Juszczak E, Brocklehurst P for the I2S2 Team

Pediatrics 2017;139:e20163703

Effect of increased enteral protein intake on growth in human milk-fed preterm infants: a randomized clinical trial

Maas C, Mathes M, Bleeker C, Vek J, Bernhard W, Wiechers C, Peter A, Poets CF, Franz AR

JAMA Pediatr 2017;171:16–22

Two-hourly versus 3-hourly feeding for very low birthweight infants: a randomised controlled trial

Ibrahim NR, Kheng TH, Nasir A, Ramli N, Foo JLK, Syed Alwi SH, Van Rostenberghe H

Arch Dis Child Fetal Neonatal Ed 2017;102:F225–F229

Prevention of vitamin K deficiency bleeding in newborn infants: a position paper by the ESPGHAN Committee on Nutrition

Mihatsch WA[1], Braegger C[2], Bronsky J[3], Campoy C[4], Domellöf M[5], Fewtrell M[6], Mis NF[7], Hojsak I[8], Hulst J[9], Indrio F[10], Lapillonne A[11], Molgaard C[12], Embleton N[13], van Goudoever J[14], ESPGHAN Committee on Nutrition

[1]Department of Pediatrics, Harlaching, Munich Municipal Hospitals, Munich, Germany; [2]Department of Pediatric Gastroenterology, University Children's Hospital, Zurich, Switzerland; [3]Department of Pediatrics, University Hospital Motol, Prague, Czech Republic; [4]Department of Pediatrics, University of Granada, Granada, Spain; [5]Department of Clinical Sciences, Pediatrics, Umea University, Umea, Sweden; [6]Childhood Nutrition Research Centre, UCL Institute of Child Health, London, UK; [7]Department of Gastroenterology, Hepatology and Nutrition, University Children's Hospital, University Medical Centre Ljubljana, Ljubljana, Slovenia; [8]University Children's Hospital Zagreb, Zagreb, Croatia; [9]Department of Pediatrics, Erasmus Medical Center, Sophia Children's Hospital, Rotterdam, The Netherlands; [10]Department of Pediatrics, University Hospital Giovanni XXIII, University Aldo Moro, Bari, Italy; [11]APHP Necker-Enfants Malades Hospital, Paris Descartes University, Paris, France and the CNRC, Baylor College of Medicine, Houston, TX, USA; [12]Department of Nutrition, Exercise and Sports, University of Copenhagen, Copenhagen, and the Hans Christian Andersen Children's Hospital, Odense University Hospital, Odense, Denmark; [13]Newcastle Neonatal Service, Newcastle Hospitals NHS Foundation Trust, Newcastle upon Tyne, UK; [14]Department of Pediatrics, VU University Medical Center, and the Department of Pediatrics, Emma Children's Hospital-AMC, Amsterdam, The Netherlands

J Pediatr Gastroenterol Nutr 2016;63:123–139

Background: Healthy newborns and infants are at risk of vitamin K deficiency bleeding (VKDB) owing to physiologically low levels of vitamin K after birth. Bleeding can be prevented by vitamin K supplementation. This position paper was published to provide a definition of the condition, to report the prevalence, review current prophylaxis practices and outcomes, and to provide recommendations.

Results: It is recommended that all newborn infants receive vitamin K prophylaxis. Possible regimens include: (1) 1 mg of vitamin K_1 by intramuscular injection at birth; or (2) 3×2 mg vitamin K_1 orally at birth, at 4–6 days and at 4–6 weeks; or (3) 2 mg vitamin K_1 orally at birth, and a weekly dose of 1 mg orally for 3 months. Parental refusal to treatment should be documented.

The optimal route is the intramuscular application, because it is efficient and assures full dose administration. Oral administration is not suitable for preterm infants, for newborns who have cholestasis or impaired intestinal absorption, or for newborns who are unwell and unable to take oral medications. Neither should it be given to infants whose mothers have taken medications that interfere with vitamin K metabolism. Parental education about the importance of vitamin K supplementation may improve compliance.

Comments Vitamin K is required for the γ-carboxylation of coagulation factors II (prothrombin), VII, IX, X, protein C, and protein S [1]. It acts as an essential cofactor for the conversion of specific peptide-bound glutamate residues to γ-carboxyglutamate residues. The abbreviation for these under-carboxylated molecules is PIVKA (proteins induced by vitamin K absence). Vitamin K does not easily cross the placenta. The fetal plasma vitamin K concentration is very low and consequently at birth, concentrations of clotting factors are low. Increased PIVKA II concentrations (>10 ng/mL), which is a biomarker of low vitamin K level, have been found in the umbilical cord blood in 10–50% of healthy term and preterm infants. Prenatal maternal vitamin K_1 supplementation does not prevent VKDB. VKDB has been classified by age of onset into early (<24 h), classic (days 1–7), and late (>1 week <6 months). Although plasma vitamin K_1 concentration is very low immediately after birth, adult levels have been recorded on days 3–4 following supplementation. Human milk vitamin K_1 concentration (median: 2.5 µg/L [0.85–9.2 µg/L]) is significantly lower than the currently available formula milk (4–25 µg/100 kcal corresponding to 24–175 µg/L). On average, daily vitamin K_1 intake of breastfed infants is <1 µg within the first 6 months of life, whereas the intake of formula-fed infants is on average up to 100 times higher. With regard to global coagulation tests such as prothrombin time, there is no significant difference between breast- and formula-fed infants. However, PIVKAs are more commonly reported in breastfed infants. Formula vitamin K_1 exceeds the recommended vitamin K intake of at least 5 µg/day. Because breastfeeding fails to provide this intake, and VKDB is much more common in unsupplemented breastfed infants, it is recommended that all infants receive some form of supplementation.

ESPGHAN CoN emphasizes in this paper that if the infant vomits or regurgitates the formulation within 1 h of administration, repeating the oral dose may be appropriate. ESPGHAN CoN also emphasizes that data from some countries suggest intramuscular application may be more effective than 3×2 mg oral prophylaxis for prevention of late VKDB. However, the more recent epidemiological data obtained from >4.5 million children show no significant difference between these 2 options with regard to the efficacy in the prevention of late VKDB. This position paper of ESPGHAN CoN will help health care providers to prevent efficiently the risk for VKDB in healthy term infants.

Long chain polyunsaturated fatty acid supplementation in infants born at term

Jasani B[1], Simmer K[2], Patole SK[3], Rao SC[4]

[1]King Edward Memorial Hospital for Women and Princess Margaret Hospital for Children, Subiaco, Australia; [2]Neonatal Care Unit, King Edward Memorial Hospital for Women and Princess Margaret Hospital for Children, Subiaco, Australia; [3]School of Paediatrics and Child Health, School of Women's and Infants' Health, University of Western Australia, King Edward Memorial Hospital, Perth, Australia; [4]Centre for Neonatal Research and Education, King Edward Memorial Hospital for Women and Princess Margaret Hospital for Children, Perth, Western Australia, Australia

Cochrane Database Syst Rev 2017;3:CD000376

This manuscript is also discussed in Chapter 4, pages 66–83.

Background: The long chain polyunsaturated fatty acids (LCPUFA) are considered vital for the maturation of the developing brain, retina, and other organs in newborn infants. Some manufacturers have added LCPUFA to IF, claiming these confer a benefit to the child's development compared with standard formula. The aim of this review was to evaluate whether adding LCPUFA to IF results in improved visual function, neurodevelopment, and physical growth.

Methods: Two review authors searched the Cochrane Central Register of Controlled Trials, Medline, Embase, the Cumulative Index to Nursing and Allied Health Literature and abstracts of the Pediatric Academic Societies. They reviewed all RCTs that dealt with the effects of LCPUFA supplements on visual function, neurodevelopment, and physical growth, conducting a meta-analysis when appropriate.

Results: A total of 31 RCTs were identified, 15 of which were included in the review ($n = 1,889$). Nine studies evaluated visual acuity, 6 by visual evoked potentials, 2 by Teller cards and one study using both. An advantage for LCPUFA was reported in 4 of these studies, but not in the remaining 5. Meta-analysis of 3 RCTs revealed significant advantage for sweep visual evoked potential acuity at 12 months (mean difference [MD] –0.15, 95% CI –0.17 to –0.13; $I^2 = 0$; 3 trials; $n = 244$), however, meta-analysis of 3 additional RCTs demonstrated no difference for visual acuity assessed with Teller cards at 12 months (MD –0.01, 95% CI –0.12 to 0.11; $I^2 = 0$; 3 trials; $n = 256$). GRADE analysis for the outcome of visual acuity implied that the overall quality of evidence was low. Eleven studies evaluated neurodevelopmental outcomes at 2 years or under. Of them, 9 studies employed Bayley Scales of Infant Development, version II (BSID-II). Benefits were demonstrated only in 2 of these studies. Meta-analysis found no significant distinction between LCPUFA and placebo groups in BSID Mental Developmental Index scores at 18 months (MD 0.06, 95% CI –2.01 to 2.14; $I^2 = 75\%$; 4 trials; $n = 661$), or in BSID Psychomotor Development Index scores at 18 months (MD 0.69, 95% CI –0.78 to 2.16; $I^2 = 61\%$; 4 trials; $n = 661$). Neither were significant differences between the 2 groups found in BSID-II scores at 12 and 24 months of age. One study described better novelty preference at 9 months. A different study reported improved problem solving at 10 months. One study used the Brunet and Lezine test for the evaluation of the developmental quotient and discovered no beneficial effects. Children who were followed until the age of 3, 6, and 9 years, in different studies, had gained no benefit by supplementation. GRADE analysis of these results revealed that the overall quality of evidence was low. Thirteen studies evaluated anthropometry; none of them exhibited a favorable or negative effect of supplementation. Meta-analysis of 5 RCTs demonstrated that the LCPUFA group had lower weight (z scores) at 12 months (MD –0.23, 95% CI –0.40 to –0.06; $I^2 = 83\%$; $n = 521$) and that the 2 groups had similar results in length and head circumference. Meta-analysis at 18 months and at 24 months found no significant differences between the 2 groups in weight, length, and head circumference. GRADE analysis of these outcomes showed that the overall quality of evidence was low.

Conclusion: The majority of RCTs demonstrated no significant influence of LCPUFA supplementation on neurodevelopmental outcomes, and only an inconsistent beneficial impact on visual acuity. For this reason, it is currently not recommended to supplement milk formula with LCPUFA.

Comments Docosahexaenoic acid (DHA) is needed for the normal development of the nervous system and the retina and accumulates in fetal brain and retina during pregnancy and in early childhood. Dietary linoleic acid (LA) and alpha-linolenic acid (ALA) can be converted by elongation of the carbon chain and the introduction of double bonds into LCPU-FAs; however, the rate of conversion of ALA to DHA in humans is low (less than 1%).

The content of arachidonic acid (AA) in human milk varies throughout the world (0.31–1.00 weight% of total fatty acids). The average AA content of human milk has been reported to be 0.47 ± 0.13 weight% of total fatty acids. DHA is the most important n-3 LC-PUFA in human milk. Depending on the region of the world and habitual dietary habits, DHA contents varying from 0.15 to 1.4 weight% of total fatty acids have been observed. Breast-fed infants accumulate more DHA in brain than infants fed formula containing ALA only and no DHA. The levels of AA and DHA in breast milk are mainly derived from maternal stores. They are, moreover, influenced by the maternal diet, in particular by its fatty acid composition and its content of trans fatty acids, and by smoking (negative for DHA). Taking into account the above-mentioned data, the European Food Safety Authority (EFSA) proposed for young infants (0–6 months) an adequate intake of 100 mg/day for DHA and 140 mg/day for AA [2].

In its Scientific Opinion on the essential composition of infant (IF) and follow-on formulae (FOF), EFSA considered, in accordance with the conclusions of the above-mentioned Cochrane review, that there is currently no conclusive evidence for any effects beyond infancy of addition of DHA to IF or FOF on the following health outcomes: neurodevelopment, visual acuity, blood pressure, and asthma [3]. However, in contrast to the Cochrane review, EFSA considered that DHA should be added to infant and FOF IF and FOF for the following reasons: (i) DHA is an essential structural component of the nervous tissue and the retina, and is involved in normal brain and visual development; (ii) the developing brain has to accumulate large amounts of DHA in the first 2 years of life; (iii) although DHA can be synthesized in the body from ALA, the intake of pre-formed DHA generally results in an erythrocyte DHA status more closely resembling that of a breast-fed infant than is achieved with ALA alone; and (iiii) although, to date, there is no convincing evidence that the addition of DHA to IF and FOF has benefits beyond infancy on any functional outcomes, there is also a lack of long-term follow-up data on specific aspects of cognitive and behavioral function from adequately powered RCTs of DHA addition to IF and FOF. Considering all of these factors, it seems prudent to provide pre-formed DHA to formula-fed infants in similar amounts as breast-fed infants.

EFSA pointed out that even though studies have shown that feeding an IF-containing DHA alone (without addition of AA) leads to lower concentrations of AA in erythrocytes compared with the consumption of control formula without DHA, no direct functional consequences have been observed in relation to growth and neurodevelopment and this lower concentration of AA in erythrocytes seems not to be associated with a decrease in concentrations of AA in the brain. The adverse effects on growth which had been reported in one RCT in pre-term infants have not been replicated in other recent trials. Therefore, EFSA considers that there is no necessity to add AA to IF even in the presence of DHA [3].

The Commission regulated regulation (EU) 2016/127 of 25 September 2015 supplementing Regulation (EU) No 609/2013 of the European Parliament and of the Council as regards the specific compositional and information requirements for IF and FOF will apply from 22 February 2020 [4]. In this regulation, it is stated that supplementation of DHA in both IF and FOF is mandatory, with a minimum content of 20 mg/100 kcal and a maximum content of 50 mg/100 kcal. Supplementation of IF and FOF with AA is not mandatory. If added, AA should not represent more than 1% of the total fat content.

Effects of infant formula with human milk oligosaccharides on growth and morbidity: a randomized multicenter trial

Puccio G[1], Alliet P[2], Cajozzo C[1], Janssens E[2], Corsello G[1], Sprenger N[5], Wernimont S[3], Egli D[4], Gosoniu L[5], Steenhout P[6]

[1]Dipartimento Materno Infantile, AOUP "Paolo Giaccone", Universita di Palermo, Palermo, Italy; [2]Department of Paediatrics, Jessa Hospital, Hasselt, Belgium; [3]Nestlé Nutrition R&D, King of Prussia, PA, USA; [4]Nestlé Nutrition, Vevey, Switzerland; [5]Nestlé Research Center, Nestec Ltd, Lausanne, Switzerland; [6]Nestlé Health Science, Epalinges, Switzerland

J Pediatr Gastroenterol Nutr 2017;64:624–631

Background: The main goal of this study was to assess the impact of the addition of 2 human milk oligosaccharides (HMOs) to infant formula on infant growth, tolerance, and morbidity.

Methods: This was a randomized trial of 2 parallel groups: the intervention group was fed with cow's milk-based infant formula with a supplement of 1.0 g/L 2'fucosyllactose (2'FL) and 0.5 g/L lacto-N-neotetraose (LNnT; test, *n* = 88) and the control group (control, *n* = 87) was fed with the same formula without supplements. Both formulae were given to healthy children from the age of 0–14 days for 6 months. All infants received standard follow-up formula without HMOs from 6 to 12 months. Primary endpoint was weight gain at age 4 months. Secondary endpoints were weight, length, body mass index, head circumference, and corresponding z scores, gastrointestinal tolerance, behavioral patterns, and morbidity during the first year of life.

Results: There was no significant difference in weight gain between the groups. Most digestive symptoms and behavioral patterns were comparable between the groups; softer stool (*p* = 0.021) and fewer nighttime wake-ups (*p* = 0.036) were found in the test group at 2 months. Infants receiving HMOs had significantly fewer events of bronchitis (*p* = 0.004–0.047) by 4 (2.3 vs. 12.6%), 6 (6.8 vs. 21.8%), and 12 months (10.2 vs. 27.6%) compared to controls (as reported by the parents); lower respiratory tract infections by 12 months (19.3 vs. 34.5%); antipyretics use at 4 months (15.9 vs. 29.9%); and antibiotics use at 6 (34.1 vs. 49.4%) and 12 months (42.0 vs. 60.9%).

Conclusion: This study demonstrated that infant formula with supplements of 2'FL and LNnT is safe and well-tolerated and does not impair growth. The association between consumption of HMO-supplemented formula and a reduction in parent-reported morbidity and medication use requires confirmation in future studies.

Comments HMOs represent approximately 20% of the total carbohydrate content of human milk and are the third largest solid component after lactose and lipids, present at concentrations of up to 20 g/L or more in colostrum [5]. Currently, approximately 150 oligosaccharide structures in human milk have been elucidated, and many more are present, at least in small quantities. The prebiotic effect of HMOs was the first function discovered. There is increasing evidence that HMOs have other functions as well, as indicated by the direct interaction of HMOs with bacterial or protozoan lectins as well as with epithelial or immune cell receptor [6]. HMOs enhance the development of the intestinal microbiota and support immune protection in breastfed infants. Although the types and concentrations of HMOs vary considerably among lactating women and over time, 2 that are commonly found in abundance in human milk are 2'FL and LNnT. This study is the first randomized, controlled trial of infant formula supplemented with both 2'FL and LNnT, that represent 37% of total HMOs in breast milk. Compared with infants fed the control formula, those fed the test formula with HMOs experienced similar age-appropriate growth, had some indication of improved GI comfort in the first few months of life, and had lower rates of parent-reported morbidities related to lower respiratory tract infections as well as antipyretic and antibiotic use. Formula intake and tolerance were not different in both groups. This study has several limitations. Gastrointestinal tolerance data were based on parent report, which are very likely to be susceptible to under- or overreporting. The use of morbidity assessments based on parent-reported symptoms/illnesses and medication use, rather than a physician-based diagnosis, is also an important limitation. Moreover, there is no information that statistical analysis took into account multiple testing. More studies on growth, prevalence of infections, and adverse events are urgently needed to confirm whether the supplementation of IF with HMOs is of interest.

First infant formula type and risk of islet autoimmunity in The Environmental Determinants of Diabetes in the Young (TEDDY) Study

Hummel S[1], Beyerlein A[1], Tamura R[2], Uusitalo U[2], Aronsson CA[3], Yang J[2], Riikonen R[4], Lernmark A[3], Rewers MJ[5], Hagopian WA[6], She JX[7], Simell OG[8], Toppari J[8, 9], Ziegler AG[1], Akolkar B[10], Krischer JP[2], Virtanen SM[4, 11], Norris JM[12] and the TEDDY Study Group

[1]Institute of Diabetes Research, Helmholtz Zentrum München, Munich, and Forschergruppe Diabetes, Klinikum rechts der Isar, Technische Universität München, Forschergruppe Diabetes e.V., Neuherberg, Germany; [2]Health Informatics Institute, Morsani College of Medicine, University of South Florida, Tampa, FL, USA; [3]Department of Clinical Sciences, Lund University/Clinical Research Centre, Skane University Hospital (SUS), Malmö, Sweden; [4]Unit of Nutrition, National Institute for Health and Welfare, Helsinki, and Faculty of Social Sciences, University of Tampere, Tampere, Finland; [5]Barbara Davis Center for Childhood Diabetes, University of Colorado Anschutz Medical Campus, Aurora, CO, USA; [6]Pacific Northwest Diabetes Research Institute, Seattle, WA, USA; [7]Center for Biotechnology and Genomic Medicine, Medical College of Georgia, Augusta University, Augusta, GA, USA; [8]Department of Pediatrics, Turku University Hospital, Turku, Finland; [9]Department of Physiology, Institute of Biomedicine, University of Turku, Turku, Finland; [10]National Institute of Diabetes and Digestive and Kidney Diseases, Bethesda, MD, USA; [11]Center for Child Health Research, University of Tampere and Tampere University Hospital, Tampere, and The Science Center of Pirkanmaa Hospital District, Tampere, Finland; [12]Department of Epidemiology, Colorado School of Public Health, University of Colorado Anschutz, USA

Diabetes Care 2017;40:398–404

Background: Several studies have examined the association between infant formulas and their impact on the risk of islet autoimmunity and type 1 diabetes (T1D), with inconsistent findings. The aim of this study was to investigate whether the introduction of infant formula based on hydrolyzed cow's milk as the first formula is related to a reduced risk of islet autoimmunity in a large prospective cohort.

Methods: The Environmental Determinants of Diabetes in the Young study follows 8,676 children at increased genetic risk for T1D. Autoantibodies to insulin, GAD65, and IA2 were routinely monitored as markers of islet autoimmunity. Information regarding infant formula feeding was elicited from questionnaires at 3 months of age.

Results: After adjustment for family history of T1D, HLA genotype, gender, country, delivery mode, breast-feeding ≥3 months, and seasonality of birth, no significant association with islet autoimmunity was observed in infants who received extensively hydrolyzed versus non-hydrolyzed cow's milk-based formula as the first formula during the first 3 months of life (adjusted hazard ratio 1.38 [95% CI 0.95–2.01]). A significantly higher risk was found when extensively hydrolyzed formula was introduced during the first 7 days of life (adjusted hazard ratio 1.57 [1.04–2.38]). Infants fed with a partially hydrolyzed or other formula as the first formula, or no formula, did not have an increased islet autoimmunity risk.

Conclusion: This study supports previous evidence implying that islet autoimmunity risk is not reduced, and may be elevated, in children at increased genetic risk for T1D who received extensively hydrolyzed rather than non-hydrolyzed cow's milk-based infant formula as the first formula.

Comments Numerous studies have examined the association between age at first exposure to cow's milk and T1D, resulting in inconsistent findings. Moreover, most prospective cohort studies showed no association between cow's milk introduction and islet autoimmunity and/or T1D risk. Most of these studies focused on whether the formulas contained cow's milk protein or not, and did not account for the use of protein hydrolysates and the degree of hydrolysis. The use of hydrolyzed cow's milk proteins has also been hypothesized to protect infants at increased T1D risk from developing islet autoimmunity [7]. However, in the Trial to Reduce IDDM in the Genetically at Risk (TRIGR), which studied 2,159 newborn infants from 15 countries, the use of an extensively hydrolyzed formula did not reduce the islet autoimmunity risk compared with conventional formula [8]. Consistent with findings from the TRIGR trial, the results of this study provide evidence that introducing an extensively hydrolyzed formula as the first infant formula does not protect children with an HLA-conferred increased risk for T1D from the development of islet autoimmunity.

Food protein-induced enterocolitis syndrome in Australia: a population-based study, 2012–2014

Mehr S[1], Frith K[1,2], Barnes EH[3], Campbell DE[1,4], on behalf of the FPIES Study Group

[1]Department of Allergy and Immunology, Children's Hospital at Westmead, Sydney, Australia; [2]Department of Immunology and Infectious Diseases, Sydney Children's Hospital, Sydney, Australia; [3]NHMRC Clinical Trials Centre, University of Sydney, Sydney, Australia; [4]Discipline of Child and Adolescent Health, Sydney University, Sydney, Australia

J Allergy Clin Immunol 2017;140:1323–1330.

Background: Food protein induced enterocolitis syndrome (FPIES) is a non-IgE-mediated allergic disorder that occurs mainly in infants and children. The aim of the study was to determine the incidence and clinical characteristics of FPIES in Australian infants.

Methods: Each month between 2012 and 2014, 1,400 participating pediatricians in Australia reported to the Australian Paediatric Surveillance Unit of new cases of acute FPIES in infants less than 24 months old.

Results: Two hundred and thirty infants were diagnosed with FPIES with an incidence of 15.4/100,000/year. The median age of the first episode and diagnosis were 5, and 7 months, respectively. Seven percent of the children had siblings with a history of FPIES, and 5% developed FPIES while feeding exclusively on breastmilk. Sixty-eight per cent of infants had a single food trigger, while 20% had 2, and 12% had ≥3 food triggers. The most frequently reported triggers were rice (45%), cow's milk (33%), and egg (12%). Fifty-one percent of the children reacted on their first known exposure. Infants with FPIES to multiple versus single food groups were younger at the first event (mean age: 4.6 vs. 5.8 months, $p = 0.001$) and more commonly had FPIES to fruits, vegetables, or both (66 vs. 21%, $p < 0.0001$). Sixty-four percent of infants with FPIES to multiple foods, which included cow's milk, also had FPIES to solid foods. Forty-two percent of infants with FPIES to fish developed a reaction to additional food groups.

Conclusion: FPIES is not uncommon and most commonly occurs as a response to a single food group. The authors suggest that infants at high risk of FPIES to multiple foods are those who present early with FPIES to fruits, vegetables, or both.

Comments The true population incidence of FPIES is unknown [9]. The only other current study on the epidemiology of FPIES, the Israeli single-center large birth cohort study by Katz et al. [10], reported a 2-year cumulative incidence of 0.34% of FPIES to cow's milk. The proportion of FPIES compared to other allergic disorders presenting at tertiary allergy clinics is estimated at about 1%. The authors of this manuscript report that rice is the most common cause of FPIES, which is in contrast to data from the US and Europe, where FPIES to cow's milk predominates and FPIES to rice represents 4–23% of all triggers. The reported US rates of FPIES to rice (19–23%) are approximately half the Australian rate. The reasons for these differences are not known, and the introduction of rice or cow's milk as the first complementary food was not an associated risk factor for the development of FPIES to either of these food triggers. Approximately two-thirds of infants in this Australian cohort had a single food trigger and 73% reacted to a single food group, which is in keeping with reports from the US and the UK. Although a causal relationship cannot be proven, this study highlights that FPIES through breast milk exposure can occur, and food proteins in breast milk appear more likely to trigger non-IgE mediated food reactions than IgE-mediated food reactions. This study also shows that FPIEs is not rare, has no sex predilection, and most commonly occurs as a response to a single food and single food group.

International consensus guidelines for the diagnosis and management of food protein-induced enterocolitis syndrome: Executive Summary – Workgroup Report of the Adverse Reactions to Foods Committee, American Academy of Allergy, Asthma and Immunology

Nowak-Wegrzyn A[1], Chehade M[2], Groetch ME[3], Spergel JM[4], Wood RA[5], Allen KJ[6], Atkins D[7], Bahna S[8], Barad AV[9], Berin C[10], Brown Whitehorn T[11], Burks WA[12], Caubet JC[13], Cianferoni C[14], Conte M[15], Davis C[16], Fiocchi A[17], Grimshaw K[19], Gupta R[20], Hofmeister B[21], Hwang JB[22], Katz Y[23], Konstantinou GN[24], Leonard SA[25], Lightdale J[26], McGhee S[27], Mehr S[28], Miceli Sopo S[29], Monti G[30], Muraro A[31], Noel SK[32], Nomura I[33], Noone S[34], Sampson HA[35], Schultz F[36], Sicherer SH[37], Thompson CC[38], Turner PJ[39], Venter C[40], Westcott-Chavez A[41], Greenhawt M[18]

[1]Division of Allergy and Immunology, Icahn School of Medicine at Mount Sinai, New York, NY, USA; [2]Eosinophilic Disorders Center, Division of Allergy and Immunology, Icahn School of Medicine at Mount Sinai, New York, NY, USA; [3]Jaffe Food Allergy, Jaffe Food Allergy Institute, Division of Allergy and Immunology, Icahn School of Medicine at Mount Sinai, New York, NY, USA; [4]Division of Allergy and Immunology, The Children's Hospital of Philadelphia, Perelman School of Medicine at University of Pennsylvania, Philadelphia, PA, USA; [5]Division of Pediatric Allergy and Immunology, Johns Hopkins University School of Medicine, Baltimore, MD, USA; [6]University of Melbourne Department of Paediatrics, Murdoch Children's Research Institute, Royal Children's Hospital Melbourne, Australia and Institute of Inflammation and Repair University of Manchester, Manchester, UK; [7]Allergy and Immunology Section, Gastrointestinal Eosinophilic Diseases Program, Children's Hospital Colorado, University of Colorado School of Medicine, Aurora, CO, USA; [8]Allergy and Immunology Section, Louisiana State University Health Sciences Center, Shreveport, LA, USA; [9]Division of Pediatric Gastroenterology, Hepatology and Nutrition Baylor Scott and White McLane Children's Medical Center and Pediatrics Texas A&M Health Sciences Center College of Medicine, Temple, TX, USA; [10]Division of Allergy and Immunology, Icahn School of Medicine at Mount Sinai, New York, NY, USA; [11]Division of Allergy and Immunology, The Children's Hospital of Philadelphia, Clinical Pediatrics Perelman School of Medicine, University of Pennsylvania, Philadelphia, PA, USA; [12]Pediatrics, University of North Carolina, Chapel Hill, NC, USA; [13]University Hospitals of Geneva, Pediatric Allergy Unit, Department of Child and Adolescent, Geneva, Switzerland; [14]Allergy and Immunology Division, Children's Hospital of Philadelphia, Perelman School of Medicine, University of Pennsylvania; Philadelphia, PA, USA; [15]Taubman Health Services Library, The University of Michigan Medical School, Ann Arbor, MI, USA; [16]Baylor College of Medicine, Houston, TX, USA; [17]Division of Allergy, Pediatric Hospital Bambino Gesu, Rome, Vatican City, Italy; [18]Pediatric Allergy Section, Children's Hospital Colorado, University of Colorado Denver School of Medicine. Denver, CO, USA;

[19]Clinical and Experimental Sciences and Human Development in Health Academic Unit, University of Southampton Faculty of Medicine and Department of Nutrition and Dietetics, Southampton's Children's Hospital, Southampton, UK; [20]Northwestern Medicine, Chicago, IL, USA and Ann and Robert H. Lurie Children's Hospital of Chicago, Chicago, IL, USA; [21]Medical Advisory Board, International FPIES Association (I-FPIES), Point Pleasant Beach, NJ, USA; [22]Department of Pediatrics, Keimyung University Dongsan Medical Center, Daegu, Korea; [23]Department of Pediatrics, Sackler School of Medicine, Tel-Aviv University, Tel-Aviv, Israel and Institute of Allergy Asthma and Immunology and Food Allergy Center, "Assaf Harofeh" Medical Center, Zerifin, Israel; [24]Department of Allergy and Clinical Immunology, 424 General Military Training Hospital, Thessaloniki, Greece and Division of Allergy and Immunology, Jaffe Food Allergy Institute, Icahn School of Medicine at Mount Sinai, New York, NY, USA; [25]Division of Pediatric Allergy and Immunology, Rady Children's Hospital San Diego, University of California, San Diego, CA, USA; [26]Pediatric Gastroenterology and Nutrition, UMass Memorial Children's Medical Center, Department of Pediatrics, University of Massachusetts Medical School, Worcester, MA, USA; [27]Division of Immunology and Allergy, Stanford University School of Medicine, Palo Alto, CA, USA; [28]Department of Allergy and Immunology, Children's Hospital at Westmead, Sydney, Australia; [29]Pediatric Allergy Unit, Department of Women and Child Health, Catholic University of Sacred Hearth, Agostino Gemelli Hospital, Rome, Italy; [30]Department of Paediatric and Adolescence Science, Regina Margherita Children's Hospital A.O.U. Citta della Salute e della Scienza, Turin, Italy; [31]Food Allergy Referral Centre Veneto Region; Department of Women and Child Health Padua, General University Hospital, Padua, Italy; [32]Emergency Medicine, University of Michigan School of Medicine, Ann Arbor, MI, USA; [33]Department of Allergy and Clinical Immunology, National Center for Child Health and Development, Tokyo, Japan; [34]Pediatric Allergy and Immunology, Jaffe Food Allergy Institute, New York, NY, USA; [35]Jaffe Food Allergy Institute, Department of Pediatrics, Icahn School of Medicine at Mount Sinai, New York, NY, USA; [36]International FPIES Association (I-FPIES), Point Pleasant Beach, NJ, USA; [37]Pediatric Allergy and Immunology, Icahn School of Medicine at Mount Sinai and Jaffe Food Allergy Institute, New York, NY, USA; [38]Division of Critical Care Medicine, Department of Pediatrics, Icahn School of Medicine at Mount Sinai, New York, NY, USA; [39]Imperial College London, Paediatric Allergy and Immunology, Imperial College Healthcare NHS Trust London, UK and Department of Pediatrics, University of Sydney, Sydney, Australia; [40]Division of Allergy and Immunology, Cincinnati Children's Hospital Medical Center, Cincinnati, OH, USA; [41]International FPIES Association I-(FPIES), Point Pleasant Beach, NJ, USA

J Allergy Clin Immunol 2017;139:1111–1126

Background: Although food protein-induced enterocolitis syndrome (FPIES) may manifest may manifest as a severe food allergy, the awareness to it is low, and there is a lack of high-quality data on the pathophysiology, diagnosis, and management of this disease. This consensus document was written by an international workgroup assembled through the Adverse Reactions to Foods Committee of the American Academy of Allergy, Asthma and Immunology and the International FPIES Association advocacy group.

Methods: A comprehensive literature review was performed by searching PubMed/Medline, Web of Science, and Embase. Excluding abstracts, a total of 879 citations were found through February 2014; of these, 110 were included. Work was divided to individual subgroup teams whose findings received feedback from all authors until a consensus was obtained. Evidence was graded according to the previously established grading system for clinical practice guidelines used by the Joint Task Force on Allergy Practice Parameters.

Results: This consensus document on FPIES comprises of the following sections: I (Definition and clinical manifestations); II (Epidemiology); III (Diagnosis of FPIES); IV (Pathophysiology of FPIES); V (Gastrointestinal manifestations of FPIES); VI (Management of acute FPIES); and VII (Nutritional management for FPIES). A list of 30 summary statements is also provided.

The following areas have been identified as having high priority for advancing the care of patients with FPIES: (1) characterize chronic FPIES; (2) establish FPIES prevalence; (3) identify FPIES risk factors; (4) validate the proposed diagnostic criteria; (5) standardize the OFC protocol and criteria for challenge positivity; (6) determine the pathophysiology of acute and chronic FPIES; (7) understand the relationship between atopy and FPIES; (8) develop noninvasive biomarkers for diagnosis and for monitoring for resolution; (9) develop therapeutic approaches to accelerate FPIES resolution; (10) determine the role of ondansetron in managing FPIES reactions; (11) determine whether extensively heated (baked) cow's milk and egg white proteins can be tolerated by children with FPIES to these foods; (12) perform systematic evaluation of the prevalence of nutrient deficiencies, poor growth, and feeding difficulties in patients with FPIES and provide guidance for preventative intervention; (13) perform longitudinal cohort studies to improve our understanding of the outcomes and the natural history of FPIES in children and adults.

Conclusion: These are the first international evidence-based guidelines to improve the diagnosis and management of patients with FPIES. These guidelines will be updated as more evidence accumulates.

Comments   This consensus document is the first international evidence-based guidelines to improve the diagnosis and management of patients with FPIES [11]. It also identifies unmet needs and future directions for research. These guidelines will be helpful for health professionals involved in FPIES diagnosis and management. Research on prevalence, pathophysiology, diagnostic markers, and future treatments is necessary to improve the care of patients with FPIES. The full report is available online as open access in this article's Online Repository at www.jacionline.org.

Complementary feeding: a position paper by the European Society for Paediatric Gastroenterology, Hepatology, and Nutrition (ESPGHAN) Committee on Nutrition

Fewtrell M[1], Bronsky J[2], Campoy C[3], Domellöf M[4], Embleton N[5], Mis NF[6], Hojsak I[7], Hulst JM[8], Indrio F[9], Lapillonne A[10], Molgaard C[11]

[1]Childhood Nutrition Research Centre, UCL Great Ormond Street Institute of Child Health, London, UK; [2]Department of Pediatrics, University Hospital Motol, Prague, Czech Republic; [3]Department of Pediatrics, University of Granada, Granada, Spain; [4]Department of Clinical Sciences, Pediatrics, Umea University, Umea, Sweden; [5]Newcastle Neonatal Service, Newcastle Hospitals NHS Trust and Newcastle University, Newcastle upon Tyne, UK; [6]Department of Gastroenterology, Hepatology and Nutrition, University Children's Hospital, University Medical Centre Ljubljana, Ljubljana, Slovenia; [7]University Children's Hospital Zagreb, Zagreb, Croatia; [8]Erasmus MC, Sophia Children's Hospital, Rotterdam, The Netherlands; [9]Ospedale Pediatrico Giovanni XXIII, University of Bari, Bari, Italy; [10]Paris Descartes University, APHP Necker-Enfants Malades Hospital, Paris, France, and the CNRC, Baylor College of Medicine, Houston, TX, USA; [11]Department of Nutrition, Exercise and Sports, University of Copenhagen, Copenhagen, and the Pediatric Nutrition Unit, Copenhagen University Hospital, Rigshospitalet, Denmark

J Pediatr Gastroenterol Nutr 2017;64:119–132

Background: This position paper discusses various aspects of complementary feeding (CF) focusing on healthy infants born at term in Europe.

Methods: The authors conducted a systematic literature search and reviewed current knowledge and practices. Based on their findings, they formulated their recommendations.

Results: Timing: Exclusive or full breastfeeding should be strongly encouraged for a minimum of 4 months (17 weeks), and exclusive or predominant breast-feeding for approximately 6 months (26 weeks) should be aimed for. Complementary foods (solids and liquids other than breast milk or infant formula) should not be introduced before 4 months but should not be withheld beyond 6 months of age. ***Content:*** Different foods of various flavors and textures including bitter-tasting green vegetables should be offered as complementary foods. Breastfeeding alongside CF is recommended. Whole cows' milk should not be provided as the main drink before the age of one year. Allergenic foods may be introduced when CF is commenced any time after 4 months. Infants who are at high risk of peanut allergy (those with severe eczema, egg allergy, or both) should have peanut introduced between 4 and 11 months, after being evaluated by a suitably trained specialist. Gluten may be introduced between 4 and 12 months, but consumption of large quantities should be avoided during the first weeks after gluten introduction and later during infancy. It is recommended that all infants receive iron-rich CF including meat products and/or iron-fortified foods. No sugar or salt should be added to CF and fruit juices or sugar-sweetened beverages should be discouraged. Vegan diets should only be applied under suitable medical or dietetic supervision, while making sure that the parents understand the importance of complying with the advice on supplementation of the diet.

Methods: Complementary food should be provided as a response to the infant's hunger and satiety queues, not as a means of comfort or as a reward.

Comments Complementary foods are important in the transition from milk feeding to family foods. The CF period is one of rapid growth and development when infants are susceptible to nutrient deficiencies and excesses, and during which there are marked changes in the diet with exposures to new foods, tastes, and feeding experiences. Little attention has been paid to the CF period, especially to the type of foods given, or whether this period of significant dietary change influences later health, development, or behavior. The relatively limited scientific evidence base is reflected in considerable variation in CF recommendations and practices between and within countries.

ESPGHAN CoN recommendations are intended for infants living in Europe, typically in relatively affluent populations with access to clean water and good healthcare. It is, however, important to ensure that advice reaches high-risk groups such as socioeconomically disadvantaged families and immigrant families, and to adapt advice for individual infants taking into account their circumstances and environment.

The purpose of this position paper is to update the position paper published by ESPGHAN CoN in 2008 [12]. New evidence has been included, particularly data from randomized controlled trials on the introduction of gluten and allergenic foods.

Timing of allergenic food introduction to the infant diet and risk of allergic or autoimmune disease. A systematic review and meta-analysis

Ierodiakonou D[1,2], Garcia-Larsen V[2], Logan A[1], Groome A[1], Cunha S[2], Chivinge J[1], Robinson Z[1], Geoghegan N[1], Jarrold K[1], Reeves T[2], Tagiyeva-Milne N[3], Nurmatov U[4], Trivella M[5], Leonardi-Bee J[6], Boyle RJ[1]

[1]Section of Paediatrics, Imperial College London, London, UK; [2]Respiratory Epidemiology, Imperial College London, London, UK; [3]Institute of Medical Sciences, University of Aberdeen, Aberdeen, Scotland; [4]University Division of Population Medicine, Cardiff University, Cardiff, Wales; [5]Centre for Statistics in Medicine, University of Oxford, Oxford, UK, [6]Division of Epidemiology and Public Health, University of Nottingham, Nottingham, UK

JAMA 2016;316:1181–1192

Background: It is unclear whether the timing of introduction of allergenic foods to the infant diet can affect the risk of allergic or autoimmune disease. The objective of this paper was to systematically review and meta-analyze evidence regarding the association between timing of allergenic food introduction during infancy and the risk of allergic or autoimmune disease.

Methods: The authors conducted a search of Medline, Embase, Web of Science, Central, and Lilacs databases between January 1946 and March 2016. The review included both observational studies and interventional trials that evaluated timing of allergenic food introduction and reported allergic or autoimmune disease during the first year of life. Data were extracted in duplicate and synthesized for meta-analysis using generic inverse variance or Mantel-Haenszel methods with a random-effects model. GRADE was used to evaluate the quality of evidence. Main outcomes and measures were wheeze, eczema, allergic rhinitis, food allergy, allergic sensitization, T1D mellitus, celiac disease, inflammatory bowel disease, autoimmune thyroid disease, and juvenile rheumatoid arthritis.

Results: The authors screened 16,289 original titles, eventually extracting data from 204 titles reporting 146 studies. There was moderate-certainty evidence from 5 trials (1,915 participants) that early egg introduction at 4–6 months was associated with a reduction in incidence of egg allergy (risk ratio 0.56; 95% CI 0.36–0.87; $I^2 = 36\%$; $p = 0.009$). The absolute risk reduction for a population of whom 5.4% had an egg allergy was 24/1,000 (95% CI 7–35 cases). There was moderate-certainty evidence from 2 studies (1,550 participants) that early peanut introduction at age 4–11 months corresponded with reduced peanut allergy (risk ratio 0.29; 95% CI 0.11–0.74; $I^2 = 66\%$; $p = 0.009$). Absolute risk reduction for a population with 2.5% risk of peanut allergy was 18/1,000 cases (95% CI 6–22 cases). Certainty of evidence was downgraded because of imprecision of effect estimates and indirectness of the populations and interventions studied. Timing of egg or peanut introduction was not associated with the risk of allergy to other foods. There was low- to very low-certainty evidence that early introduction of fish correlated with reduced allergic sensitization and rhinitis. There was high-certainty evidence that timing of gluten introduction was not associated with the risk of celiac disease, and that timing of initiation of other allergenic foods was not associated with other outcomes.

Conclusion: It was found that early egg or peanut introduction to infants' diets carries a lower risk of developing egg or peanut allergy.

Comments   Food allergy is a difficult disorder without a cure or treatment and with negative health and economic outcomes [13]. Prevention of disease occurrence and related negative consequences through an inexpensive intervention is of high interest. Infant feeding guidelines have moved away from advising parents to delay the introduction of allergenic food, but most guidelines do not yet advise early feeding of such foods. The evidence base for a relationship between early allergenic food introduction and food allergy to the same food was limited to a relatively small number of studies and events and was only statistically significant for egg and peanut.

The findings of this review are consistent with a large body of experimental data in various animal models in which early enteral antigen exposure is established as effective for preventing allergic sensitization to the same antigen. Oral tolerance in humans appears to be antigen specific, with no data showing early introduction of one allergenic food influences the development of allergy to a different allergenic food. In contrast to egg and peanut allergies, this review found that oral tolerance was not relevant to celiac disease, suggesting that the findings may not be generalizable beyond food allergy mediated by IgE antibodies. These data suggest that current guidelines that do not advise early introduction of allergenic foods may need to be revised.

Early introduction of foods may not be a panacea to address the food allergy epidemic. In addition, it is not clear that it is the specific early introduction of an allergenic food that renders immunological protection, rather than the accompanying increased diversity in the diet that occurs concomitantly.

Complementary feeding at 4 versus 6 months of age for preterm infants born at less than 34 weeks of gestation: a randomised, open-label, multicentre trial

Gupta S[1], Agarwal R[1], Aggarwal KC[2], Chellani H[2], Duggal A[1,3], Arya S[2], Bhatia S[1,3], Sankar MJ[1], Sreenivas V[1], Jain V[1], Gupta AK[1], Deorari AK[1], Paul VK[1]; Investigators of the CF trial

[1]All India Institute of Medical Sciences, Delhi, India; [2]Vardhman Mahavir Medical College and Associated Safdarjung Hospital, New Delhi, India; [3]Kasturba Hospital, Delhi, India

Lancet Glob Health 2017;5:e501–e511

Background: Evidence on the preferable time to of complementary feeding (CF) in preterm infants is lacking. The influence of initiation of CF at 4 months versus 6 months (corrected age) on weight for age at the age of one year corrected age in preterm infants born at less than 34 weeks of gestation was therefore examined.

Methods: This was an open-label, randomized trial, in which infants born at less than 34 weeks of gestation with no major malformation were enrolled from 3 centers in India. Eligible infants were followed from birth and were randomly assigned at 4 months corrected age to begin CF at 4 months corrected age (4 month group), or to continue with milk feeding and initiate CF at 6 months corrected age (6 month group). Groups were stratified according to gestation (30 weeks or under, and 31–33 weeks). All participants received standard iron supplementation. Primary outcome was weight for age z-score at 12 months corrected age (WAZ_{12}) based on WHO Multicentre Growth Reference Study growth standards. Analyses were by intention to treat.

Results: A total of 403 infants were randomly assigned: 206 to initiate CF at 4 months and 197 to initiate CF at 6 months. Twenty-two infants in the 4-month group (4 deaths, 2 withdrawals, 16 lost to follow-up) and 8 infants in the 6-month group (2 deaths, 6 lost to follow-up) were excluded from analysis of primary outcome. No difference in WAZ_{12} was found among the 2 groups: –1.6 (SD 1.2) in the 4-month group versus –1.6 (SD 1.3) in the 6 month group. A higher rate of hospital admissions was reported in the 4-month group compared with the 6-month group: 2.5 episodes/100 infant-months versus 1.4 episodes/100 infant-months, respectively (incidence rate ratio 1.8, 95% CI 1.0–3.1, $p = 0.03$).

Conclusion: Early versus late introduction of CF in preterm infants did not affect WAZ_{12}. However, a higher rate of hospital admission in the 4-month group supports the introduction of CF at 6 months rather than at 4 months of corrected age, in infants born before 34 weeks of gestation.

Comments   Very few data are available with respect to the optimal time of initiation of CF in preterm infants who are at a much higher risk of postnatal growth restriction than full-term infants [14]. Extrapolating or not the recommendation for full-term infants to initiate CF at 6 months of age to preterm infants depends on 2 major questions: what does 6 months refer to in a preterm infant – chronological (postnatal) age or corrected age? Healthcare providers generally use corrected age for monitoring the physical growth and development of preterm infants. In addition, if it is assumed that 6 months refers to the corrected age, should these infants not start CF earlier than full-term infants? Preterm infants have higher energy requirements compared with full-term infants, and it is not known how long in infancy milk feeds alone (breast milk or formula) are sufficient to meet their requirements. Most complementary foods provide higher caloric density compared with milk feeds. Therefore, an early introduction of CF in preterm infants than is recommended for full-term infants might improve their growth.

This study shows that early initiation of CF at 4 month compared with 6 months of corrected age does not improve the growth of preterm infants at corrected age of 12 months. It also does not result in a difference in developmental outcomes, body composition, bone mineralization, and any marker for metabolic syndrome like insulin resistance, lipid profile, and blood pressure in infancy. Rather, early initiation of CF at 4 months corrected age increases the risk of hospital admission due to concurrent morbidities, predominantly diarrhoea and lower tract respiratory infections. In both groups, dietary patterns remained poor and body iron stores remained depleted despite iron supplementation until 12 months of corrected age. This may be related to the vegetarian diet received by most infants, with co-consumption of phytates and oxalates, and low vitamin C intake, and/or to infrequent practice of delayed umbilical cord clamping.

This well-designed randomized study is of high relevance for preterm infants from low-income populations. However, conclusions cannot be generalized to high income countries mainly because of high mortality rate, different conditions of hygiene and environment, and vegetarian dietary practices. High-quality studies on the timing of CF in preterm infants are urgently needed in high-income populations.

A micronutrient-fortified young-child formula improves the iron and vitamin D status of healthy young European children: a randomized, double-blind controlled trial

Akkermans MD[1], Eussen SRBM[2], van der Horst-Graat JM[2], van Elburg RM[2, 3], van Goudoever JB[3, 4], Brus F[1]

[1]Department of Pediatrics, Juliana Children's Hospital/Haga Teaching Hospital, The Hague, Netherlands; [2]Danone Nutricia Research, Utrecht, Netherlands; [3]Department of Pediatrics, Emma Children's Hospital/Academic Medical Center, Amsterdam, Netherlands; [4]Department of Pediatrics, VU University Medical Center, Amsterdam, Netherlands

Am J Clin Nutr 2017;105:391–399

Background: Many young European children develop iron deficiency (ID) and vitamin D deficiency (VDD) due to insufficient dietary intakes and poor compliance to vitamin D supplementation. The aim of this study was to evaluate the effect of a micronutrient-fortified young-child formula (YCF) on the iron and vitamin D status of young European children.

Methods: This randomized, double-blind controlled trial, was conducted in Western Europe (Germany, the Netherlands, and England) from October 2012 to September 2014. Healthy children aged 1–3 years received either YCF (1.2 mg Fe/100 mL; 1.7 μg vitamin D/100 mL) or non-fortified cow's milk (CM; 0.02 mg Fe/100 mL; no vitamin D) for 20 weeks. The primary and secondary outcomes were change from baseline in serum ferritin (SF) and 25-hydroxyvitamin D (25[OH]D), respectively. ID was defined as SF <12 μg/L in the absence of infection (high-sensitivity C-reactive protein <10 mg/L) and VDD as 25(OH)D <50 nmol/L. Statistical adjustments were made in intention-to-treat analyses for sex, country, age, baseline micronutrient status, and micronutrient intake from food and supplements (and sun exposure for vitamin D outcomes).

Results: Three hundred and eighteen children, mainly Caucasian, participated in this study. The difference between the groups in the SF and 25(OH)D status from baseline was 6.6 μg/L (95% CI 1.4–11.7 μg/L; $p = 0.013$) and 16.4 nmol/L (95% CI 9.5–21.4 nmol/L; $p < 0.001$), respectively. The risk of developing ID (OR 0.42; 95% CI 0.18–0.95; $p = 0.036$) and VDD (OR 0.22; 95% CI 0.01–0.51; $p < 0.001$) after the intervention was lower in the YCF group than in the CM group.

Conclusion: Consumption of micronutrient-fortified YCF daily for 20 weeks preserved the iron status, lowered the risk of ID, and improved vitamin D status in healthy young children in Western Europe.

Comments   Despite national nutritional recommendations, ID and VDD are among the most common micronutrient deficiencies in young children living in industrialized countries. Compliance to the use of iron and/or vitamin D supplements seems to be low. Therefore, fortification of commonly used products has been suggested. Milk is a popular source for delivering fortification in non-breastfed infants because of its wide availability and acceptance (infant formula from 0 to 6 months; follow-on formula from 6 to 12 months; YCF in young children from 1 to 3 years).

In the study, the estimated mean ± SEM change in SF concentration from baseline was –4.9 ± 2.2 μg/L for the CM group and +1.7 ± 2.4 μg/L for the YCF group. The estimated mean ± SEM change in 25(OH)D concentration from baseline was –7.2 ± 2.5 nmol/L for the CM group and +9.2 ± 2.8 nmol/L for the YCF group. At baseline, 8.2% of the YCF group and 5.6% of the CM group were iron- and vitamin D-deficient. These prevalence rates increased in the CM group to 15.3% and decreased for YCF users to 4.0% after 20 weeks of study product intake. There were no statistical differences in anthropometric data, stool pattern, and occurrence of overall adverse events between the YCF and the CM groups. This well-designed study is the first randomized, double-blind controlled trial assessing the impact of YCF on both the iron and vitamin D status. The daily consumption of YCF for 20 weeks was shown to preserve the iron status and improve vitamin D status. The authors conclude that the use of YCF may be an effective and practical strategy for preventing both ID and VDD in young European children.

In its Scientific Opinion on nutrient requirements and dietary intakes of infants and young children in the European Union [2], EFSA pointed out that dietary intakes of ALA, DHA, iron, vitamin D, and iodine (in some European countries) are low in infants and young children living in Europe. Particular attention should be paid to ensuring an appropriate supply of ALA, DHA, iron, vitamin D, and iodine in infants and young children with inadequate or at-risk of inadequate status of these nutrients.

There is as yet no European legislation covering the composition and main characteristics of young-child formulae. In comparison with CM, YCF currently marketed in the

European Union contain more ALA, DHA (if added), iron, and vitamin D but similar amounts of iodine. The median content of these nutrients in YCF is within the range of permitted concentrations in FOF and, except for iron, also in IF. Fortified formulae, including YCF, are one of the several means to increase n-3 PUFA, iron, vitamin D, and iodine intakes in infants and young children living in Europe with inadequate or at-risk of inadequate status of these nutrients. However, other means, such as fortified cow's milk, fortified cereals and cereal-based foods, supplements or the early introduction of meat and fish into CF and their continued regular consumption, are alternatives to increase intakes of these nutrients. The selection of the appropriate form and vehicle through which these nutrients are provided in the diet will depend on national dietary habits, health authorities, the regulatory context, and caregivers' preference. At the present time, no unique role of YCF with respect to the provision of critical nutrients in the diet of infants and young children living in Europe can be identified, so that they cannot be considered as a necessity to satisfy the nutritional requirements of young children.

To conclude, this very interesting study shows the usefulness of YCF to prevent ID and VDD in young children. It was not designed to demonstrate that it is the only means to do it. There is a controversy as to whether a specific regulation on YCF marketed in the EU is needed. An easy alternative to such a regulation is the use of FOF between 1 and 3 years of age as one of the means to compensate for lower intake of iron, vitamin D, DHA, ALA, and iodine in this at-risk population.

Preterm Infants

Randomized trial of two doses of vitamin D3 in preterm infants <32 weeks: dose impact on achieving desired serum 25(OH)D3 in a NICU population

Anderson-Berry A[1], Thoene M[2], Wagner J[3], Lyden E[4], Jones G[5], Kaufmann M[5], Van Ormer M[1], Hanson C[6]

[1]Department of Pediatrics, University of Nebraska Medical Center, Omaha, NE, USA; [2]Neonatal Intensive Care Unit, The Nebraska Medical Center, Omaha, NE, USA; [3]CHI Health, Omaha, NE, USA; [4]College of Public Health, University of Nebraska Medical Center, Omaha, NE, USA; [5]Department of Biomedical and Molecular Sciences, Queen's University, Kingston, Ontario, Canada; [6]Division of Medical Nutrition Education, School of Allied Health Professions, University of Nebraska Medical Center, Omaha, NE, USA

PLoS One 2017;12:e0185950

Background: Various different recommendations for vitamin D supplementation for preterm neonates exist. However, evidence regarding the effect of the different doses on outcomes of these infants is insufficient.

Objective: The aim of this double-blind randomized controlled study was to evaluate 2 different doses of serum 25(OH)D$_3$ concentration on a preterm population and assess the impact on Neonatal Intensive Care Unit (NICU) outcomes.

Design: Out of 369 infants assessed for eligibility, 32 infants born at 24–32 weeks gestation were prospectively randomized into 2 groups: one received 400 IU/day and the other 800 IU/day of vitamin D_3 supplementation. Serum $25(OH)D_3$ levels were measured once in 4 weeks. The Wilcoxon signed rank test was used to compare serum levels of $25(OH)D_3$ at 4 weeks and at each subsequent time point. A p value of <0.05 was considered statistically significant.

Results: Serum $25(OH)D_3$ levels at birth were 41.9 and 42.9 nmol/L for infants in the 400 IU group and 800 IU group, respectively ($p = 0.86$). A significant correlation was found between cord $25(OH)$ D_3 concentrations and gestational age ($r = 0.40$, $p = 0.04$). The study demonstrated a significant improvement in $25(OH)D_3$ status in the higher dose ($p = 0.048$). Infants in the 400 IU group were more prone to have dual energy X-ray absorptiometry bone density measurements below the 10th percentile. This difference was found to be significant (56 vs. 16%, $p = 0.04$). There was a trend towards improved linear growth in the 800 IU group.

Conclusions: The results suggest that there is a need for a daily supplementation of 800 IU of vitamin D for infants <32 weeks cared for in the NICU.

Comments For years, controversy exists regarding the optimal dose of vitamin D administered to preterm infants. Daily dose recommendations vary from 200 to 1,000 IU/day. The wide variation is due to a lack of solid evidence what is best for preterm infants. Similarly, the target plasma concentrations are not defined consistently either. ESPGHAN recommends $25(OH)D_3$ serum levels above 80 nmol/L, whereas other societies recommend serum levels >50 nmol/L while all aim at an outcome that involves bone health [15–17]. Altogether, this leads to uncertainty as to how much should be given to preterm infants, especially very preterm infants. The present study tries to provide an answer to both questions. The limited number of infants studied prevents any firm conclusions, but does show that 800 IU/day results in higher $25(OH)D_3$ serum levels as expected. More importantly, a lower number of infants face levels below 50 nmol/L while the higher intakes were associated with a lower number of infants with a reduced bone mineral density. Safety is of course an issue, but no infants were observed with any sign of toxicity. Therefore, this study adds to the growing evidence that additional vitamin D intakes of 800 IU/day are needed for preterm infants.

Follow-up of a randomized trial on post-discharge nutrition in preterm-born children at age 8 years

Ruys CA[1], van de Lagemaat M[1], Finken MJ[2], Lafeber HN[1]

Departments of [1]Pediatrics/Neonatology and [2]Pediatric Endocrinology, VU University Medical Center, Amsterdam, The Netherlands

Am J Clin Nutr 2017;106:549–558

Background: Preterm-born infants are subject to adverse outcomes. Therefore, research in this population is focused not only on their survival but also on the improvement of their long-term outcomes. There is still a debate regarding the optimal post-discharge nutrition of preterm infants. This research follows a previous randomized controlled study that showed that preterm-born infants, fed an isocaloric protein- and mineral-enriched post-discharge formula (PDF) from term to 6-months corrected age (CA), gained more lean mass than did those fed with standard term formula (TF).

Objective: The goal of this follow-up study was to compare alterations in body size, body composition, and metabolic health at 8 years of age, in preterm-born children who were fed with either PDF or TF from term age until 6-month CA.

Design: Seventy-nine of 152 children (52%) who completed the original trial were included in this follow-up study at the age of 8-years. Anthropometry was measured by standard methods. Body composition, including fat mass, lean mass, bone mineral content, and bone mineral density, was ascertained by dual-energy X-ray absorptiometry. Blood pressure was measured in the supine position by using an automatic device. Blood samples for various metabolic variables were drawn after an overnight fast. Nutritional habits were recorded by the parents using a 3-day nutritional diary.

Results: The authors did not find any differences in body size, body composition, bone variables, and metabolic status at age of 8-years between those who fed PDF and those fed TF.

Conclusions: In this long-term follow-up study, the authors showed that the positive impact of PDF at 6-month CA was no longer evident at the age of 8 years, but this could also be attributed to attrition. They recommend that future studies focusing on nutritional interventions in the pre- and post-discharge period regard these interventions as a continuum rather than as separate entities.

Comments The objective of nutritional management of neonatologist should be to mimic intra-uterine growth and obtain a functional outcome comparable to those infants born at term [15]. That preterm infants have higher nutrient requirements than their term equivalents is obvious but until what period following birth one should provide these preterm born infants and children with additional nutrients is unclear. This study adds to the conclusion of the recent (2016) Cochrane review that the role of post-discharge formula is questionable [18]. Only when term formula was compared to preterm formula, an effect on anthropometric values was noticed. Important is that most studies are of questionable quality. Also, this publication suffers from a high loss to follow-up number, which is not surprising as the follow-up lasted up to 8 years.

Recent studies show that direct and adequate nutrition management in the first week of life reduces the longitudinal standard deviation-loss in weight, height, and head circumference [19]. This policy reduces the need for catch-up growth, which is associated with long-term consequences with regard to blood pressure, cardiovascular biomarkers, and insulin sensitivity. Altogether, this emphasizes the importance of an adequate early nutritional supply to accomplish adequate postnatal growth and healthy neurocognitive and metabolic development [20].

Supplemental iodide for preterm infants and developmental outcomes at 2 years: an RCT

Williams FLR[1], Ogston S[1], Hume R[1], Watson J[1], Stanbury K[2], Willatts P[3], Boelen A[4], Juszczak E[2], Brocklehurst P[5] for the I2S2 Team

[1]Division of Population Health Sciences, Ninewells Hospital and Medical School, University of Dundee, Dundee, UK; [2]Nuffield Department of Population Health, NPEU Clinical Trials Unit, National Perinatal Epidemiology Unit, University of Oxford, Oxford, UK; [3]Department of Psychology, University of Dundee, Dundee, UK: [4]Neonatal Screening Laboratory, Laboratory of Endocrinology, Academic Medical Centre, Amsterdam, The Netherlands; [5]Institute for Women's Health, University College London, London, UK

Pediatrics 2017;139:e20163703

Background: Thyroid hormone is essential for normal brain development in utero and for the first 2 years of life. Preterm infants are particularly vulnerable to iodide insufficiency and thyroid dysfunction. The European guidelines for preterm enteral iodide intake is 11–55 µg/kg/day. However, it has been suggested that the enteral intake for healthy preterm infants should be at least 30–40 and 1 µg/kg/day for parenteral intake. The aim of this study was to determine whether, compared with placebo, iodide supplementation of preterm infants improves neurodevelopmental outcomes at 2 years.

Methods: In this randomized controlled trial, iodide supplementation or placebo was given to infants born before 31 weeks' gestation. Trial solutions of sodium iodide or sodium chloride were given at 30 µg/kg/day beginning within 42 h of birth until 34 weeks' gestational age. Thyroxine, thyrotropin, and thyroid-binding globulin levels were measured in whole blood drawn on postnatal days 7, 14, 28, and at 34 weeks' gestational age. The primary outcome was neurodevelopmental status at 2 years of age, evaluated using the BSID–III. The primary analyses were by intention-to-treat, and data were presented also for survivors.

Results: Out of 1,273 infants who were enrolled from 21 UK neonatal units, 997 infants survived (498 intervention and 499 placebo) and underwent neurodevelopmental evaluation. No significant differences were found between the intervention and placebo groups in the primary outcome: MD cognitive score, –0.34, 95% CI –2.57 to 1.89; motor composite score, 0.21, 95% CI –2.23 to 2.65; and language composite score, –0.05, 95% CI –2.48 to 2.39. There was a weak correlation between iodide supplementation and hypothyroxinemia in the language composite score and 1 subtest score.

Conclusions: Results from this study revealed no overall benefit of iodide supplementation on neurodevelopment of preterm infants at 2 years of age.

Comments Iodide requirements for preterm infants are difficult to assess. Iodide is pivotal for thyroid hormone synthesis, and preterm infants are frequently facing transient hypothyroxinemia [21] because of iodide deficiency [22, 23]. Both iodide and T4 supplementation has been studied. Only 1 study of thyroxine supplementation in preterm infants included long-term neurodevelopmental outcome and the results were equivocal [24]. In that study, infants receiving T4 supplementation (compared with placebo) scored 18 points higher than those aged 2 years on the Bayley-II cognitive component, but only if they were <27 weeks' gestation; supplemented infants born ≥27 weeks scored 10 points lower than non-supplemented infants. Subsequent follow-up at 5.7 and 10 years confirmed these findings [25, 26]. Clinical treatment with thyroxine has increased 2.6-fold in neonates born <27 weeks' gestation [27], so the above mentioned study was very necessary. Huge numbers of infants were studied in this pragmatic trial, with a clear primary outcome. The study group concluded that iodide supplementation does not provide a benefit. For now, that is an appropriate conclusion and no preterm infant that has no sign of hypothyroidism should be supplemented until longer term data are available and more discriminating test can be used than the BSID-III score.

Effect of increased enteral protein intake on growth in human milk-fed preterm infants: A randomized clinical trial

Maas C[1], Mathes M[1], Bleeker C[1], Vek J[1], Bernhard W[1], Wiechers C[1], Peter A[3–5], Poets CF[1], Franz AR[1, 2]

[1]University Children's Hospital, Eberhard-Karls University, Tuebingen, Germany; [2]Center for Pediatric Clinical Studies, University Children's Hospital, Eberhard-Karls University, Tuebingen, Germany; [3]Division of Endocrinology, Diabetology, Vascular Medicine, Nephrology and Clinical Chemistry, and Pathobiochemistry, Department of Internal Medicine IV, University of Tuebingen, Tuebingen, Germany; [4]Institute of Diabetes Research and Metabolic Diseases (IDM) of the Helmholtz Center Munich, University of Tuebingen, Tuebingen, Germany; [5]German Center for Diabetes Research (DZD), Muenchen-Neuherberg, Germany

JAMA Pediatr 2017;171:16–22

Background: The optimal dose of enteral protein intake for very preterm infants has not yet been determined. It has been suggested that the amount of protein supplied in currently available commercial fortifiers is not sufficient. Furthermore, both intra- and inter-individual variabilities of human milk protein and energy content may be partially responsible for inadequate early postnatal growth.

Objective: To evaluate the influence of different amounts of enteral protein supplementation on growth in preterm infants fed with human milk.

Methods: This randomized, and partially blinded study, was conducted in a neonatal tertiary referral center in Germany between October 2012 and October 2014. Infants born at gestational age of under 32 weeks and of birth weight below 1,500 g were recruited. All analyses were conducted in an intention-to-treat population. At a postnatal age of 6–8 days, participants were randomly assigned either a lower-protein supplementation (1 g of bovine protein in 100 mL of breast milk; $n = 30$) or a higher-protein supplementation (study fortifier of 1.8 g of bovine protein/100 mL of breast milk [$n = 15$], or individualized high-protein supplementation based on protein and fat content of administered breast milk [$n = 15$]). Supplementations were given for 30–57 days and until definite discharge planning. Primary outcome was weight gain (g/kg/day) from birth to the end of intervention.

Results: Sixty participants were enrolled in the study (35% of 173 eligible infants). Both groups were similar in demographic characteristics and hospital courses. The median gestational age at birth was 29.9 weeks. The higher protein group consumed 0.6 g/kg/day (0.4–0.7 g/kg/day) more protein than the lower protein group ($p < 0.001$), while the proportion of total enteral feeding volume provided as breast milk was similar between the groups. Nevertheless, there was no difference in the primary outcome between the groups: weight gain was 16.3 g/kg/day (15.4–17.1 g/kg/day) in the lower protein group, and 16.0 g/kg/day (15.1–16.9 g/kg/day) in the higher protein group ($p = 0.70$). Head circumference and lower leg longitudinal growth were also comparable.

Conclusions: An increase of 0.6 g protein/kg/day to a mean intake of 4.3 g/kg/day did not improve the growth rate of very preterm infants with a median birth weight of 1,200 g. This may point to the optimal amount of protein required for enhancing growth in this population.

Comments Have we reached the upper limit with regard to protein supplementation at around 3.5–4.0 g/kg/day for preterm infants? Yet another trial that shows no benefit of supplementation of additional protein as 2 were published recently as well [28, 29]. Although studies to date are very few in number, they point towards the same direction, although Miller et al. found a small effect on the head circumference growth. Could it be due to the quality of the supplement used? Not likely as weight gain is restricted by the first limiting essential amino acid if enough energy is provided. As both trials provided enough energy, the supplement is derived from bovine milk protein, the likelihood that all essential amino acids meet the requirement for optimal growth is very high. Thus, we can conclude that either other factors than essential amino acids are responsible for the ceiling effect or that the growth rates obtained in these studies are reaching intrauterine rates which is the maximum. Of course, it is possible to reach higher weight gain rates by providing more energy, but that is at the expense of additional fat accumulation. The early and adequate use of parenteral nutrition reduces the need for catch-up growth, so probably the intake of enteral protein should not exceed 4.0 g/kg/day under normal conditions.

Two-hourly versus 3-hourly feeding for very low birthweight infants: a randomised controlled trial

Ibrahim NR[1], Kheng TH[1], Nasir A[1], Ramli N[1], Foo JLK[2], Syed Alwi SH[2], Van Rostenberghe H[1] [1]Department of Paediatrics, School of Medical Sciences, Universiti Sains Malaysia, Kubang Kerian, Kelantan, Malaysia; [2]Department of Paediatrics, Hospital Sultanah Nur Zahirah, Kuala Terengganu, Terengganu, Malaysia

Arch Dis Child Fetal Neonatal Ed 2017;102:F225–F229

Background and aim: The practice as to the time intervals at which enteral feeding is administered varies in different intensive care units. The aim of the study was to establish whether feeding with 2- versus 3-hourly intervals in very low birthweight infants has an effect on the time at which full enteral feeding is achieved, and on the regaining of birth weight.

Methods: A total of 144 preterm infants, from 2 regional tertiary neonatal intensive care units in Malaysia, with gestational age less than 35 weeks and birth weight between 1 and 1.5 kg participated in the study and were assigned to 2 groups of 72 subjects each: 2- or 3-hourly interval feeding after randomization.

The primary outcome was time to achieve full enteral feeding ($\geq$100 mL/kg/day) and secondary outcomes were the time to regain birth weight, episodes of feeding intolerance, peak serum bilirubin levels, duration of phototherapy, episodes of necrotizing enterocolitis, nosocomial sepsis, and gastro-esophageal reflux.

Results: The mean time to full enteral feeding was 11.3 days in the 3-hourly group and 10.2 days in the 2-hourly group (MD 1.1 days; 95% CI –0.4 to 2.5; p = 0.14). Infants in the 3-hourly group regained birth weight earlier than those in the 2-hourly group (12.9 vs. 14.8 days, p = 0.04). Additional significant results were not found in subgroup analyses. There was no difference in adverse events between the groups.

Conclusions: Time to full enteral feeding was similar in infants fed every 2 h, and those fed every 3 h. The authors suggest that if these findings are confirmed by additional studies, a 3-hourly interval could be a preferable interval, in terms of reducing the work load of the NICU staff.

Comments A pragmatic trial, as a follow-up to another recently published trial compared semi-continuous feeding versus a 3-hourly feeding. Although definitions were slightly different (here, full enteral feeding was defined as 100 mL/kg/day; in the RCT performed by Rövekamp-Abels et al. [30], the definition of full enteral feeding was set at 120 mL/kg/day), both studies did not find a statistically significant difference in time to reach full enteral nutrition. Noteworthy is that the time needed to reach this primary endpoint was approximately half in the Rövekamp-Abels study, while the definition was more strict, that is, a higher volume was needed to meet the criterion "full enteral nutrition." This shows the difference in feeding schedules for many units between Asia and Europe and was a topic in a recent Cochrane review [31]. From the results of 9 trials, with approximately 1,000 preterm infants participating, the reviewers concluded that advancing enteral feed volumes at daily increments of 30–40 mL/kg (compared to 15–24 mL/kg) does not increase the risk of NEC or death in VLBW infants. Advancing the volume of enteral feeds at slow rates results in several days of delay in establishing full enteral feeds and increases the risk of invasive infection.

Of interest is a sub analysis of the Ibrahim manuscript. As Rövekamp-Abels concluded, larger infants seem to benefit more from bolus feeding than smaller infants. The applicability of these findings to extremely preterm, extremely low birth weight, or growth-restricted infants is limited. Further randomized controlled trials in these populations may be warranted to resolve this uncertainty.

References

1 McNinch A: Vitamin K deficiency bleeding: early history and recent trends in the United Kingdom. Early Hum Dev 2010;86(suppl 1):63–65.

2 EFSA NDA Panel (EFSA Panel on Dietetic Products, Nutrition and Allergies), 2013. Scientific Opinion on nutrient requirements and dietary intakes of infants and young children in the European Union. EFSA J 2013;11:3408.

3 EFSA NDA Panel (EFSA Panel on Dietetic Products, Nutrition and Allergies), 2014. Scientific Opinion on the essential composition of infant and follow-on formulae. EFSA J 2014;12:3760.

4 Commission Delegated Regulation (EU) 2016/127 of 25 September 2015 supplementing Regulation (EU) No 609/2013 of the European Parliament and of the Council as regards the specific compositional and information requirements for infant formula and follow-on formula and as regards requirements on information relating to infant and young child feeding. Official Journal of the European Union. 2.2.2016. L 25/1. 29 pages.

5 Thurl S, Munzert M, Boehm G, Matthews C, Stahl B: Systematic review of the concentrations of oligosaccharides in human milk. Nutr Rev 2017;75:920–933.

6 Bode L: The functional biology of human milk oligosaccharides. Early Hum Dev 2015;91:619–622.

7 Knip M, Virtanen SM, Seppä K, Ilonen J, Savilahti E, Vaarala O, et al; Finnish TRIGR Study Group: Dietary intervention in infancy and later signs of beta-cell autoimmunity. N Engl J Med 2010;363:1900–1908.

8 Knip M, Akerblom HK, Becker D, Dosch HM, Dupre J, Fraser W, et al; TRIGR Study Group: Hydrolyzed infant formula and early β-cell autoimmunity: a randomized clinical trial. JAMA 2014;311:2279–2287.

9 Leonard SA, Nowak-Wegrzyn A: Food protein-induced enterocolitis syndrome. Pediatr Clin North Am 2015;62:1463–1477.

10 Katz Y, Goldberg MR, Rajuan N, Cohen A, Leshno M: The prevalence and natural course of food protein-induced enterocolitis syndrome to cow's milk: a large-scale, prospective population-based study. J Allergy Clin immunol 2011;127:647–653.e1–e3.

11 Boyce JA, Assa'ad A, Burks AW, Jones SM, Sampson HA, Wood RA, et al: Guidelines for the diagnosis and management of food allergy in the United States: summary of the NIAID-sponsored Expert Panel Report. J Allergy Clin Immunol 2010;126:1105–1118.

12 Agostoni C, Decsi T, Fewtrell M, Goulet O, Kolacek S, Koletzko B, et al; ESPGHAN Committee on Nutrition: Complementary feeding: a commentary by the ESPGHAN Committee on Nutrition. J Pediatr Gastroenterol Nutr 2008;46:99–110.

13 Jones SM, Burks AW: Food allergy. N Engl J Med 2017;377:1168–1176.

14 Embleton ND: Early Nutrition and Later Outcomes in Preterm Infants; in Shamir R, Turck D, Phillip M (eds): Nutrition and Growth. Basel, Karger, 2013, pp 26–32.

15 Agostoni C, Buonocore G, Carnielli VP, De Curtis M, Darmaun D, Decsi T, Domellöf M, Embleton ND, Fusch C, Genzel-Boroviczeny O, et al: Enteral nutrient supply for preterm infants: commentary from the European Society for Paediatric Gastroenterology, Hepatology and Nutrition Committee on Nutrition. J Pediatr Gastroenterol Nutr 2010;50:85–91.

16 Abrams SA, Committee on Nutrition: Calcium and vitamin d requirements of enterally fed preterm infants. Pediatrics 2013;131:e1676–e1683.

17 WHO: Guidelines on Optimal Feeding of Low Birth-Weight Infants in Low- and Middle-Income Countries. Geneva, 2011.

18 Young L, Embleton ND, McGuire W: Nutrient-enriched formula versus standard formula for preterm infants following hospital discharge. Cochrane Database Syst Rev 2016;12:CD004696.

19 Roelants JA, Vlaardingerbroek H, van den Akker CHP, de Jonge RCJ, van Goudoever JB, Vermeulen MJ: Two-year follow-up of a randomized controlled nutrition intervention trial in very low-birth-weight infants. JPEN J Parenter Enteral Nutr 2016: 148607116678196.

20 Ong KK, Kennedy K, Castaneda Gutierrez E, Forsyth S, Godfrey K, Koletzko B, Latulippe ME, Ozanne SE, Rueda R, Schoemaker MH, et al: Postnatal growth in preterm infants and later health outcomes: a systematic review. Acta Paediatr 2015;104:974–986.

21 Williams FL, Mires GJ, Barnett C, Ogston SA, van Toor H, Visser TJ, Hume R; Scottish Preterm Thyroid Group: Transient hypothyroxinemia in preterm infants: the role of cord sera thyroid hormone levels adjusted for prenatal and intrapartum factors. J Clin Endocrinol Metab 2005;90:4599–4606.

22 Ibrahim M, de Escobar GM, Visser TJ, Duran S, van Toor H, Strachan J, Williams FL, Hume R: Iodine deficiency associated with parenteral nutrition in extreme preterm infants. Arch Dis Child Fetal Neonatal Ed 2003;88:F56–F57.

23 Ares S, Escobar-Morreale HF, Quero J, Duran S, Presas MJ, Herruzo R, Morreale de Escobar G: Neonatal hypothyroxinemia: effects of iodine intake and premature birth. J Clin Endocrinol Metab 1997;82: 1704–1712.

24 van Wassenaer AG, Kok JH, de Vijlder JJ, Briet JM, Smit BJ, Tamminga P, van Baar A, Dekker FW, Vulsma T: Effects of thyroxine supplementation on neurologic development in infants born at less than 30 weeks' gestation. N Engl J Med 1997;336:21–26.

25 Briet JM, van Wassenaer AG, Dekker FW, de Vijlder JJ, van Baar A, Kok JH: Neonatal thyroxine supplementation in very preterm children: developmental outcome evaluated at early school age. Pediatrics 2001;107:712–718.

26 van Wassenaer AG, Westera J, Houtzager BA, Kok JH: Ten-year follow-up of children born at <30 weeks' gestational age supplemented with thyroxine in the neonatal period in a randomized, controlled trial. Pediatrics 2005;116:e613–e618.

27 Linn M, Yoder BA, Clark RH: Increasing supplemental thyroid hormone use among premature infants born at 23 to 32 weeks' gestation. Am J Perinatol 2010;27:731–735.

28 Bellagamba MP, Carmenati E, D'Ascenzo R, Malatesta M, Spagnoli C, Biagetti C, Burattini I, Carnielli VP: One extra gram of protein to preterm infants from birth to 1,800 g: a single-blinded randomized clinical trial. J Pediatr Gastroenterol Nutr 2016;62: 879–884.

29 Miller J, Makrides M, Gibson RA, McPhee AJ, Stanford TE, Morris S, Ryan P, Collins CT: Effect of increasing protein content of human milk fortifier on growth in preterm infants born at <31 wk gestation: a randomized controlled trial. Am J Clin Nutr 2012; 95:648–655.

30 Rovekamp-Abels LW, Hogewind-Schoonenboom JE, de Wijs-Meijler DP, Maduro MD, Jansen-van der Weide MC, van Goudoever JB, Hulst JM: Intermittent bolus or semicontinuous feeding for preterm infants? J Pediatr Gastroenterol Nutr 2015;61:659–664.

31 Morgan J, Young L, McGuire W: Slow advancement of enteral feed volumes to prevent necrotising enterocolitis in very low birth weight infants. Cochrane Database Syst Rev 2015;2:CD001241.

Koletzko B, Shamir R, Turck D, Phillip M (eds): Nutrition and Growth: Yearbook 2018.
World Rev Nutr Diet. Basel, Karger, 2018, vol 117, pp 66–83 (DOI: 10.1159/000484500)

Cognition

Carlo Agostoni · Silvia Bettocchi

Pediatric Clinic, Department of Clinical Sciences and Community Health, University of Milan, Fondazione IRCCS Ospedale Maggiore Policlinico, Milan, Italy

Gestation and early childhood are crucial periods in child neurodevelopment and are critically dependent on several factors.

Nutritional deficiencies may affect infant health, in particular brain development.

Maternal nutritional status during pregnancy and breastfeeding and nutrients intake during infancy and childhood should be decided towards ensuring the genetic potential of brain growth and optimal functional outcomes through all the life-course.

Several studies regarding the interaction of nutrients with neurocognitive performance of children have been performed. Available results are heterogeneous, while institutions are calling for newer evidence to substantiate recommendations on dietary intakes and/or specific nutrient integration.

The microbial community represents the last promising frontier of the links between diet and development, and investigators are increasingly exploring this topic. Accordingly, a *healthy* commensal gut microbiota is crucial for a physiological neurocognitive development (but the definition of *healthy* is still under investigation, extending through the whole alimentary trait and beyond). New research should be devoted to understanding the patterns of gut microbial colonization and the mechanisms by which they may influence brain pathways.

This chapter comprehended a selection of recent articles including clinical trials, observational studies or reviews, in the area of nutrition and cognition. All articles have been selected from literature from July 1, 2016 to June 30, 2017 and fall into 4 categories: (1) long-chain polyunsaturated fatty acid (LCPUFA) gestation and lactation, (2) Micronutrients and neurodevelopment (3), Microbiome, and (4), a brief paragraph of Miscellanea.

Papers have been summarized and comments are included following the summaries.

Key articles reviewed for this chapter

LCPUFA

Long chain polyunsaturated fatty acid supplementation in infants born at term

Jasani B, Simmer K, Patole SK, Rao SC

Cochrane Database of Syst Rev 2017;3:CD000376

Prenatal supplementation with DHA improves attention at 5 y of age: a randomized controlled trial

Ramakrishnan U, Gonzalez-Casanova I, Schnaas L, DiGirolamo A, Quezada AD, Pallo BC, Hao W, Neufeld LM, Rivera JA, Stein AD, Martorell R

Am J Clin Nutr 2016;104:1075–1082

Breastfeeding, polyunsaturated fatty acid levels in colostrum and child intelligence quotient at age 5–6 years

Bernard JY, Armand M, Peyre H, Garcia C, Forhan A, De Agostini M, Charles M-A, Heude B; EDEN Mother-Child Cohort Study Group (Etude des Déterminants pré- et postnatals précoces du développement et de la santé de l'Enfant)

J Pediatr 2017;183:43–50

Association between maternal intake of n-6 to n-3 fatty acid ratio during pregnancy and infant neurodevelopment at 6 months of age: results of the MOCEH cohort study

Kim H, Kim H, Lee E, Kim Y, Ha EH, Chang N

Nutr J 2017;16:23

Docosahexaenoic acid and neurodevelopmental outcomes of term infants

Meldrum S, Simmer K

Ann Nutr Metab 2016;69(suppl 1):23–28

Impact of the n-6:n-3 long-chain PUFA ratio during pregnancy and lactation on offspring neurodevelopment: 5-year follow-up of a randomized controlled trial

Brei C, Stecher L, Brunner S, Ensenauer R, Heinen F, Wagner PD, Hermsdörfer J, Hauner H

Eur J Clin Nutr 2017;71:1114–1120

Micronutrients

Assessing infant cognitive development after prenatal iodine supplementation

Bell MA, Ross AP, Goodman G

Am J Clin Nutr 2016;104(suppl):928S–934S

Multiple biomarkers of maternal Iron predict infant cognitive outcomes

Thomas DG, Kennedy TS, Colaizzi J, Aubuchon-Endsley N, Grant S, Stoecker B, Duell E

Dev Neuropsychol 2017;42:146–159

Impact of maternal selenium status on infant outcome during the first 6 months of life

Varsi K, Bolann B, Torsvik I, Eik TC, Høl PJ, Bjørke-Monsen AL

Nutrients 2017;9:486

Maternal multiple micronutrient supplementation and other biomedical and socioenvironmental influences on children's cognition at age 9–12 years in Indonesia: follow-up of the SUMMIT randomised trial

Prado EL, Sebayang SK, Apriatni M, Adawiyah SR, Hidayati N, Islamiyah A, Siddiq S, Harefa B, Lum J, Alcock KJ, Ullman MT, Muadz H, Shankar AH

Lancet Glob Health 2017;5:e217–e228

Microbiome

Gut microbiota: a potential regulator of neurodevelopment

Tognini P

Front Cell Neurosci 2017;11:25

The central nervous system and the gut microbiome

Sharon G, Sampson TR, Geschwind DH, Mazmanian SK

Cell 2016;167:915–932

Miscellanea

Neurodevelopment: the impact of nutrition and inflammation during early to middle childhood in low-resource settings

John CC, Black MM, Nelson III CA

Pediatrics 2017;139(suppl 1):S59–S71

Assessment of neurodevelopment, nutrition, and inflammation from fetal life to adolescence in low-resource settings

Suchdev PS, Boivin MJ, Forsyth BW, Georgieff MK, Guerrant RL, Nelson III CA

Pediatrics 2017;139(suppl 1):S23–S37

Association between maternal nutritional status in pregnancy and offspring cognitive function during childhood and adolescence: a systematic review

Veena SR, Gale CR, Krishnaveni GV, Kehoe SH, Srinivasan K, Fall CH

BMC Pregnancy Childbirth 2016;16:220

Maternal dietary patterns during pregnancy and intelligence quotients in the offspring at 8 years of age: findings from the ALSPAC cohort

Freitas Vilela AA, Pearson RM, Emmett P, Heron J, Smith AD, Emond A, Hibbeln JR, Castro MB, Kac G

Matern Child Nutr 2018;14:e12431

From neuro-pigments to neural efficiency: the relationship between retinal carotenoids and behavioral and neuroelectric indices of cognitive control in childhood

Walk AM, Khan NA, Barnett SM, Raine LB, Kramer AF, Cohen NJ, Moulton CJ, Renzi-Hammond LM, Hammond BR, Hillman CH

Int J Psychophysiol 2017;118:1–8

LCPUFA

Long chain polyunsaturated fatty acid supplementation in infants born at term

Jasani B[1], Simmer K[2], Patole SK[3], Rao SC[4]

[1]King Edward Memorial Hospital for Women and Princess Margaret Hospital for Children, Subiaco, Australia; [2]Neonatal Care Unit, King Edward Memorial Hospital for Women and Princess Margaret Hospital for Children, Subiaco, Australia; [3]School of Paediatrics and Child Health, School of Women's and Infants' Health, University of Western Australia, King Edward Memorial Hospital, Perth, Australia; [4]Centre for Neonatal Research and Education, King Edward Memorial Hospital for Women and Princess Margaret Hospital for Children, Perth, Western Australia, Australia

Cochrane Database of Syst Rev 2017;3:CD000376

This manuscript is also discussed in Chapter 3, pages 39–65.

Objectives: To assess the effectiveness and safety of LCPUFA supply on formula in full-term infants, focusing on neurodevelopment and physical growth.

Methods: Findings on the effect of LCPUFA supplementation in infants born at term on their cognitive function has been reviewed.

Two authors reviewed all randomized controlled trials (RCTs) in the current literature independently.

Main Results: Thirty-one RCTs were found and 15 of these have been included in the review (*n* = 1,889). All trials enrolled infants of ≥37 weeks' gestation at birth. Recommendations as to whether infant formula should be supplemented with LCPUFA are controversial.

Conclusions: Conclusive findings on the impact of milk administration with LCPUFA in full-term infants are still lacking.

Comments   This Cochrane review included 15 RCTs that evaluated the safety and the effectiveness of supplementing formula with LCPUFA for visual acuity, neurodevelopmental outcomes, and physical growth in term infants. The overall quality of evidence was low and there is inconclusive evidence to support or refute LCPUFA supplementation of infant milk formula. For this reason, a recommendation of this common practice cannot be drowned. A cost-benefit analysis on this issue becomes mandatory before concluding, as ever, "Well-conducted RCTs with adequate and reliable sample size are still needed."

Prenatal supplementation with DHA improves attention at 5 y of age: a randomized controlled trial

Ramakrishnan U[1], Gonzalez-Casanova I[1], Schnaas L[2], DiGirolamo A[3], Quezada AD[4], Pallo BC[1], Hao W[1], Neufeld LM[5], Rivera JA[4], Stein AD[1], Martorell R[1]

[1]Hubert Department of Global Health, Rollins School of Public Health, Emory University, Atlanta, GA; [2]Division of Public Health, National Institute of Perinatology, Mexico City, Mexico; [3]Center of Excellence for Children's Behavioral Health, Georgia Health Policy Center, Georgia State University, Atlanta, GA; [4]Health and Nutrition Research Center, National Institute of Public Health, Cuernavaca, Mexico; and [5]Global Alliance for Improved Nutrition, Geneva, Switzerland

Am J Clin Nutr 2016;104:1075–1082

Background: Very few (if any) well-designed RCTs have assessed the influence of prenatal docosahexaenoic acid (DHA) supplementation on offspring brain growth and function at long term through childhood.

Methods: Neurodevelopment, behavioral and executive functioning, including attention have been assessed at 5 years of age in 797 children of Mexican women in a randomized controlled trial of prenatal DHA supplementation. In the present study 1,094 mothers were randomized to receive a total dose of 400 mg of DHA/day or a placebo from 18 to 22 weeks of gestation until birth. Measures of child cognition, behavior, and attention have been collected with the use of specific scales of intelligence and tests. Information about parental, environmental influence and social status have been assessed.

Results: No significant differences between intervention and control groups across a range of maternal and child characteristics have been found. Prenatal DHA supplementation had no overall impact on measures of cognitive functioning at 5 years of age, but interacted with the environmental effect on infant cognition in later life. Moreover, a potential effect of DHA supplementation during pregnancy on sustained attention in children at 5 years of age has been shown.

Conclusions: DHA supply in prenatal age may play a role in the development of global cognition, not limited with a better sustained attention in preschool children.

Comments The objective of this randomized control trial was to define whether DHA supply during pregnancy improves child cognition and performance on an objective measure of attention at 5 years of age.

Results obtained in this study confirm this relationship and authors suggest that an adequate maternal DHA supplementation during gestation and breastfeeding represents the key to ensure optimal levels in children and consequently to obtain better outcomes, considering also the interactions with the environmental conditions. The long-term meaning remains to be interpreted.

Breastfeeding, polyunsaturated fatty acid levels in colostrum and child intelligence quotient at age 5–6 years

Bernard JY[1,2], Armand M[3], Peyre H[4,5], Garcia C[3], Forhan A[1,2], De Agostini M[1,2], Charles M-A[1,2,6], Heude B[1,2]; EDEN Mother-Child Cohort Study Group (Etude des Déterminants pré- et postnatals précoces du développement et de la santé de l'Enfant)

[1]Epidemiology and Biostatistics Sorbonne Paris Cité Centre (CRESS), Developmental Origins of Health and Disease (ORCHAD) Team, Inserm, Villejuif, France; [2]Paris Descartes University, France; [3]Centre National de la Recherche Scientifique, Center for Magnetic Resonance in Biology and Medicine, Aix-Marseille Université, Marseille, France; [4]Laboratory of Cognitive Sciences and Psycholinguistics (École Normale Supérieure, École des Hautes Études en Sciences Sociales, Centre National de la Recherche Scientifique), École Normale Supérieure, PSL Research University, Paris, France; [5]Child and Adolescent Psychiatry Unit, Assistance Publique – Hôpitaux de Paris, Robert Debré Hospital, Paris, France and [6]Fondation PremUP, Paris, France

J Pediatr 2017;183:43–50

Background: Omega-6 and omega-3 polyunsaturated fatty acid (PUFA), naturally present in human milk, take part in the brain growth during infancy. Available data on the association between PUFA in breast milk and Intelligence Quotient (IQ) of children at 5–6 years of age are discordant.
Methods: A total of 2,002 women were recruited in the study and were tested with their offspring, by using self-administered questionnaires and medical records to obtain general information about feeding habits, alcohol consumption, smoking status, education level, household income. Anthropometric measurements and 5 mL of colostrum were also collected and analyzed. The IQ of 1,080 children at 5–6 years of age was estimated by the use of the Wechsler Preschool and Primary Scale of Intelligence-III.
Results: Breastfeeding was associated with higher IQs than no performed lactation practice, but only in models unadjusted for confounders and demographics, while any breastfeeding duration was associated with both full and verbal IQ. As for associations with PUFAs, low linoleic (LA) and high DHA in colostrum were associated with lower IQs compared with high DHA and low LA and DHA together.
Conclusions: Associations were found between duration of lactation and PUFA levels in colostrum, with children's IQs at 5–6 years of age.

Comments   This observational study reports the follow-up of a preview survey performed in the French Etude des Déterminants pré- et postnatals précoces du développement et de la santé de l'Enfant mother-child cohort. They found a moderate positive association between lactation duration and colostrum PUFA levels with child's IQ at age 5–6 years, but, taken the observations together, only a further support to the current recommendations to promote breastfeeding can be derived.

Indeed, the observations suggest a positive effect of high DHA and low LA levels in colostrum, respectively, on IQ development. Nevertheless, many factors (either genetic and/or environmental), could be at the origin of the differences in the fatty acid pattern.

Association between maternal intake of n-6 to n-3 fatty acid ratio during pregnancy and infant neurodevelopment at 6 months of age: results of the MOCEH cohort study

Kim H[1], Kim H[1], Lee E[2], Kim Y[3], Ha E-H[4], Chang N[1]

[1]Department of Nutritional Science and Food Management, Ewha Womans University, Seoul, South Korea; [2]Department of Nutrition Consultation, Seoul National University Hospital, Healthcare System Gangnam Center, Seoul, South Korea; [3]Department of Child Psychiatry, National Center for Child and Adolescent Psychiatry, Seoul National University Hospital, Seoul, South Korea; [4]Department of Occupational and Environmental Medicine, Ewha Womans University, College of Medicine, Seoul, South Korea

Nutr J 2017;16:23

Background: It is largely agreed that LCPUFAs have an important impact on brain growth during infancy.

Furthermore, it is recommended to ensure not only an optimal LCPUFAs intake but also a correct fatty acid ratio of n-6 to n-3 (n-6/n-3 PUFAs) through mothers' diet.

Methods: This study was conducted by using available data from a community-based prospective birth cohort study: Mothers' and Children's Environmental Health. A total of 960 pregnant women were enrolled in the study. The investigators tested them and subsequently their infants at 6 months of age to obtain general and specific information about nutrient intakes, food habits, and consumption by the use of questionnaires and recall methods. They calculated the maternal intakes ratio of n-6/n-3 PUFAs and linoleic acid/α-linolenic acid (LA/ALA).

Furthermore, they assessed infant cognitive and motor development by the Korean Bayley scales of infant development edition II (BSID-II) including the mental developmental index (MDI) and the psychomotor developmental index (PDI).

Results: After adjustment for confounders, negative associations were found between maternal dietary n-6/n-3 PUFA ratios and the MDI and the PDI, and between LA/ALA ratio and the MDI and the PDI in infants at 6 months of age.

The risk to observe infants with delayed performance tended to increase with increasing values of the maternal n-6/n-3 PUFA and LA/ALA ratios, respectively.

Conclusions: The authors found a significant negative association of maternal intakes of both n-6/n-3 PUFAs and LA/ALA with infant neurodevelopment and motor function at 6 months of age, but no association between absolute amounts of total n-6, n-3, LA, and ALA and the investigated developmental parameters.

Comments   The investigators suggest to ensure an adequate n-6, n-3, LA and ALA intake in the context of a well-balanced maternal diet during gestation, where balance between fatty acid families could have more impactful than absolute amounts. These recommendations may result in an improvement of global nutritional status of pregnant women that positively influences infant neurodevelopment.

Docosahexaenoic acid and neurodevelopmental outcomes of term infants

Meldrum S, Simmer K

Centre for Neonatal Research and Education, University of Western Australia, Subiaco, WA, Australia

Ann Nutr Metab 2016;69(suppl 1):23–28

Review: Seafood, fish oil, and breast milk naturally contain DHA, a fatty acid involved in the normal brain growth. DHA intake of infants occurs predominantly through placental transfer during gestation and through dietary intake after birth. In Western countries, these needs are often not completely covered. Many observational studies and randomized clinical trials focused on DHA supply during pregnancy and/or lactation and cognitive development. Findings do not recommend DHA supplementation of healthy pregnant and lactating women, nor healthy infants because of the presence of controversial and inconclusive evidence about this interaction.

Comments This welcome review, authored by a Cochrane reviewer of PUFA effects, finally underlines once more the "original sin" of research on the role of dietary PUFAs in the first ages of life, from intrauterine life to lactation. Thus, study trials suffer from large degrees of heterogeneity between the studies (dosage, intervention period, outcomes). Future efforts should be able to identify responders to dietary DHA before establishing dose and timing of interventions.

Impact of the n-6:n-3 long-chain PUFA ratio during pregnancy and lactation on offspring neurodevelopment: 5-year follow-up of a randomized controlled trial

Brei C[1], Stecher L[1], Brunner S[1], Ensenauer R[2, 3], Heinen F[4], Wagner PD[5], Hermsdörfer J[5], Hauner H[1, 6]

[1]Else Kröner-Fresenius Center for Nutritional Medicine, Klinikum rechts der Isar, Technische Universität München, Munich, Germany; [2]Department of General Pediatrics, Neonatology and Pediatric Cardiology, Experimental Pediatrics and Metabolism, University Children's Hospital, Heinrich Heine University Düsseldorf, Düsseldorf, Germany; [3]Research Center, Dr. von Hauner Children's Hospital, Ludwig-Maximilians-Universität München, Munich, Germany; [4]Department of Pediatric Neurology and Developmental Medicine, Dr von Hauner Children's Hospital, Ludwig-Maximilians-Universität München, Munich, Germany; [5]Department of Sport and Health Sciences, Institute of Human Movement Science, Technische Universität München, Munich, Germany; [6]ZIEL – Institute for Food and Health, Nutritional Medicine Unit, Technische Universität München, Freising, Germany

Eur J Clin Nutr 2017;71:1114–1120

Background: LCPUFAs are essential for infant neurodevelopment. Current findings about the role of n-3 LCPUFA supplementation during gestation on children cognition are inconsistent.
Methods: In this analysis, 208 healthy pregnant women from Germany were randomized to receive a total dose of 1,020 mg DHA +180 mg EPA +9 mg vitamin E from the 15th week until 4 months postpartum as well as dietary counseling aimed at lowering arachidonic acid intake (intervention group) or to follow a healthy diet during pregnancy according to the German guidelines (control group). Brain growth and function of their children were assessed using a global questionnaire, and a specific hand movement test, and also cord blood LCPUFAs were analyzed. Subsequently, the association with these outcomes was evaluated.

Results: Results obtained show neither positive nor negative effects on neurodevelopment of children at preschool age, just inconsistent and not-significant associations, with a change in the n-6:n-3 LCPUFA ratio during gestation.

Comments The investigators analyzed data from the INFAT study, and in this article they present secondary results to describe if a reduced n-6:n-3 fatty acid ratio in diet of women during pre and post-natal feeding has positive effects on cognitive function of their children at 4 and 5 years of age. Even if it is widely accepted that LCPUFAs play an important role in brain and neural development, current findings, regarding the impact of n-3 supply during pregnancy on child neurodevelopment, are inconsistent. It is worth nothing that the present study has looked at the association between LCPUFAs longer chain derivatives and outcomes, differently than other studies previously mentioned that focused on the ratios between the 2 PUFA precursors. Once more, heterogeneity creates more confusion, that is, at the end, there are no recommendations concerning the present practice, at least in theory.

Micronutrients

Assessing infant cognitive development after prenatal iodine supplementation

Bell MA[1], Ross AP[1], Goodman G[2]

[1]Department of Psychology, Virginia Tech, Blacksburg, VA, USA; [2]Human Health Risk Research, Seattle, WA, USA

Am J Clin Nutr 2016;104(suppl):928S–934S

Review: The investigators first evaluated the prenatal neurodevelopment and the timing of thyroid hormone action on specific brain systems associated with iodine deficiency. Later, they focused their attention on the infant cognitive development and function in prenatal supplementation studies conducted in regions of mild to moderate iodine deficiency.

The authors performed a PubMed search on studies of prenatal iodine supplementation, and they identified the use of these global tests; BSID and Brunet-Lézine scale.

They considered neurodevelopmental outcomes associated with maternal thyroid hormone and maternal iodine status during prenatal period, and tried to evaluate whether specialized cognitive tasks might be more useful than the BSID for assessing the potential effects of prenatal iodine supplementation on cognitive functions.

Comments It is largely accepted that an optimal iodine status is crucial for early-life neurodevelopment. There are inconclusive findings on the effects of prenatal iodine supplementation on the cognitive outcomes of children in regions of mild to moderate iodine deficiency. Infant visual attention might be a sensitive measure of infant outcomes because during the prenatal period, the visual attention abilities are sensitive to thyroid hormone. For this reason, the authors propose the use of this measure to improve the reliability of neurodevelopmental and cognitive performance, particularly in regions of mild to moderate iodine deficiency. Multidisciplinary collaborations between scientists would improve research on prenatal iodine supplementation.

Multiple biomarkers of maternal iron predict infant cognitive outcomes

Thomas DG[1], Kennedy TS[2], Colaizzi J[1], Aubuchon-Endsley N[3], Grant S[4], Stoecker B[2], Duell E[5]

[1]Department of Psychology, Oklahoma State University, Stillwater, OK, USA; [2]Department of Nutritional Sciences, Oklahoma State University, Stillwater, OK, USA; [3]Department of Psychology, Idaho State University, Pocatello, ID, USA; [4]Department of Psychology, Hope College, Holland, MI, USA; [5]Laureate Institute for Brain Research, Tulsa, OK, USA

Dev Neuropsychol 2017;42:146–159

Background: Iron deficiency is common in several countries in the developing world and also in industrialized nations, especially in women.

Methods: The aim of the present observational study was to evaluate the role of the following maternal iron biomarkers: Hemoglobin (Hgb), ferritin, soluble transferrin receptors (sTfR), the ratio of sTfR to ferritin (sTfR:ferritin ratio) and plasma iron, on infant neurocognitive performance. A total of 132 women and their infants were enrolled in the study; mothers completed a demographic form and the Pregnancy Risk Assessment Monitoring System Phase 5 Core Questionnaire at the 3-month visit. Weight and length were measured and infant body mass index (BMI) z-scores were calculated. Venous blood samples were collected and several cognitive tests were performed.

Results: At 9 months, maternal plasma iron correlated positively with novelty preference (memory) and maternal Hgb correlated positively with sustained attention. Furthermore, a negative correlation has been found between plasma iron and neural response variability tertile change.

Conclusions: An improved maternal tissue-level iron may have a role on brain growth and function of children, even in a well-nourished sample. Most studies have been conducted so far in populations with poor iron nutrition, therefore, now other studies in well-nourished countries are needed.

Comments The authors found inconsistent associations between maternal Hgb and cognitive function. They showed an association with only a single domain, novelty quotient. However, considering multiple iron biomarkers, associations with multiple domains were found. Consequently, we conclude that newer studies with more biologically available pools of iron and specific cognitive domains should be analyzed to enlarge our knowledge on this interesting topic, particularly from well-developed, Western countries.

Impact of maternal selenium status on infant outcome during the first 6 months of life

Varsi K[1], Bolann B[1, 2], Torsvik I[3], Eik TCR[1], Høl PJ[4], Bjørke-Monsen AL[1]

[1]Laboratory of Clinical Biochemistry, Haukeland University Hospital, Bergen, Norway; [2]Department of Clinical Science, Faculty of Medicine and Dentistry, University of Bergen, Bergen, Norway; [3]Department of Pediatrics, Haukeland University Hospital, Bergen, Norway; [4]Department of Clinical Medicine, Faculty of Medicine and Dentistry, University of Bergen, Bergen, Norway

Nutrients 2017;9:486

Background: Selenium is relevant for immune and brain development in the first stages of life.

Methods: One hundred fourteen healthy pregnant, 158 healthy, never-pregnant women and their offspring were included in this observational study, performed in Norway. Associations between maternal selenium levels in blood and breast milk on infant brain growth and function during the first 6 months of life were studied. Clinical data (body weight, nutrition) and the parental question-naire Ages and Stages were used to evaluate infant neurodevelopment besides selenium analysis of blood and breast milk of mothers.

Results: A negative association between maternal selenium level (≤0.90 µmol/L) at 18 weeks of gestation and infant neurodevelopment was found. At 36 weeks of pregnancy, an association between maternal selenium level ≤0.78 µmol/L and an increased risk of infant infection during the first 6 weeks of life has been reported too.

Conclusions: Intervention studies are needed to substantiate the hypothesis raised by the observations.

Comments   It is widely accepted that selenium is a crucial component for human metabolism. Interest in selenium metabolism has been raised also by the proposed narrow range of recommended dosages for a beneficial effect. Scant experimental data suggest selenium deficiency might negatively affect infant health, in particular immune and brain functions.

Blood selenium levels decreased significantly during pregnancy ($p < 0.001$), then their levels increased postpartum and remained unchanged from 6 weeks to 6 months. Furthermore, maternal selenium status directly influences the levels of this element in breast milk, as partly expected.

The investigators suggest the opportunity to keep into account a selenium cutoff of 0.90 µmol/L in pregnancy week 18 and 0.78 µmol/L in pregnancy week 36. Intervention studies are needed to obtain specific selenium levels to improve maternal status and infant outcomes.

Maternal multiple micronutrient supplementation and other biomedical and socioenvironmental influences on children's cognition at age 9–12 years in Indonesia: follow-up of the SUMMIT randomised trial

Prado EL[1,2], Sebayang SK[1], Apriatni M[1], Adawiyah SR[1], Hidayati N[1], Islamiyah A[1], Siddiq S[1], Harefa B[1], Lum J[3], Alcock KJ[4], Ullman MT[5], Muadz H[1,6], Shankar AH[1,7]

[1]Summit Institute of Development, Mataram, Nusa Tenggara Barat, Indonesia; [2]Department of Nutrition, University of California Davis, Davis, CA, USA; [3]School of Psychology, Deakin University, Melbourne, VIC, Australia; [4]Psychology Department, Lancaster University, Bailrigg, Lancaster, UK; [5]Department of Neuroscience, Georgetown University, Washington, DC, USA; [6]Center for Research on Language and Culture, University of Mataram, Mataram, Nusa Tenggara Barat, Indonesia; [7]Department of Nutrition, Harvard TH Chan Boston, MA, USA

Lancet Glob Health 2017;5:e217–e228

Background: Several factors (biomedical and socioenvironmental) play an important role on the brain growth and function.

Methods: The authors performed a follow-up of a double-blind, cluster-randomised trial, named Supplementation with Multiple Micronutrients Intervention Trial in Indonesia, in which 262 government midwives were randomly assigned to distribute either iron and folic acid (IFA) or multiple micronutrients (MMN) to pregnant women enrolled in the study.

The IFA capsule contained 30 mg iron as ferrous fumarate and 400 µg folic acid. The MMN capsule contained the same amounts of IFA, plus 800.0 µg retinol, 200.0 IU vitamin D, 10.0 mg vitamin E, 70.0 mg ascorbic acid, 1.4 mg vitamin B1, 1.4 mg vitamin B2 (riboflavin), 18.0 mg niacin,

1.9 mg vitamin B6, 1.6 μg vitamin B12, 15.0 mg zinc, 2.0 mg copper, 65.0 μg selenium, and 150.0 μg iodine. Then 3,068 children were selected for cognitive assessment: nurturing and stimulation from the environment and maternal depression were evaluated using specific tests. Children were tested on cognition and motor performance at local schools and medical information were collected.

Results: Participants were divided into 3 groups: a randomly selected representative sample, one from undernourished and one from anemic mothers. In the representative sample and in children of anemic women, tests respectively on procedural memory and on intellectual ability showed positive coefficients of MMN versus IFA.

Overall, 18 out of 21 estimates were positive, indicating that the MMN group scored consistently higher than the IFA group.

The regression coefficients for all variables showed that socioenvironmental determinants had stronger associations with school-age cognitive, motor, and socioemotional determinants, as compared with the biomedical factors (22 of 35 coefficients were significant versus 8 of 56). The significant difference in these proportions ($p < 0.0001$) indicated a more consistent impact of socioenvironmental factors.

Conclusions: Results showed higher scores in the MMN group than in the IFA group, indicating a strong impact of maternal MMN supplementation on neurodevelopment and cognitive performance in the offspring, later in life. Furthermore, a preponderant positive role of socioenvironmental determinants on cognitive outcomes of children has been found.

Comments The aim of this study was to examine the effects of a multimineral-multivitamin supplementation, MMN, versus iron plus folate, IFA, only and the impact of biomedical and socioenvironmental factors on child neurocognitive, motor, and socioemotional development.

The authors found a strong link between maternal MMN supplementation and a better cognitive performance of their children compared to IFA, and a stronger impact of socioenvironmental determinants on child neurodevelopment. Therefore, the primary take-home message concerns the necessity of implementing interventions on socioenvironmental determinants, including those to reduce maternal depression and improve educational levels.

Microbiome

Gut microbiota: a potential regulator of neurodevelopment

Tognini P

Sassone-Corsi Laboratory, Center for Epigenetics and Metabolism, Department of Biological Chemistry, University of California Irvine, Irvine, CA, USA

Front Cell Neurosci 2017;11:25

Review: More evidence is accumulating that environmental influences during early life may profoundly affect brain development and function later in life. The neurodevelopmental process starts during pregnancy and protracts after birth. The first years of postnatal life represent a time of rapid changes in brain structure and function, where neuronal circuits are particularly sensitive to environmental inputs. It is becoming clear that there is a link between microbiome and neurodevelopment.

After birth, the newborn is colonized with a community of microbes. This postnatal microbial colonization may contribute to developmental programming of epithelial barrier function, gut homeostasis, and angiogenesis, as well as the development and function of the gut immune system. Moreover, this process seems to influence the early-life programming of brain circuits involved in the control of stress response, motor activity, anxiety-like behavior, and cognitive function.

Comments   This review considered studies investigating the relationship between brain and gut microbiota. It is clear that several factors play a role on infant gut colonization. Recent evidence has shown comorbidity between neurodevelopmental diseases and the gastrointestinal trait denoting a possible intersection of dysbiosis and neurological illness, that needs to be clarified. The authors considered probiotics, prebiotics, and dietary manipulations as a promising way to improve brain development and function in early childhood.

The central nervous system and the gut microbiome

Sharon G[1], Sampson TR[1], Geschwind DH[2-5], Mazmanian SK[1]

[1]Division of Biology and Biological Engineering, California Institute of Technology, Pasadena, CA, USA; [2]Program in Neurobehavioral Genetics, Semel Institute, and Program in Neurogenetics; [3]Department of Neurology, David Geffen School of Medicine, University of California, Los Angeles, Los Angeles, CA, USA; [4]Center for Autism Treatment and Research, Semel Institute, David Geffen School of Medicine, University of California, Los Angeles, Los Angeles, CA, USA; [5]Department of Human Genetics, David Geffen School of Medicine, University of California, Los Angeles, Los Angeles, CA, USA

Cell 2016;167:915–932

Review: The influence of microbial community on brain growth has been suggested by several observations. During neurodevelopment, many factors (pre- and post-natally) are involved in this complex process. One of these factors is represented by molecular signal from the gut. In this review, the interaction of the microbiota with central nervous system is widely discussed.

Comments   An increasing number of studies hypothesize that perturbations of maternal gut microorganisms may influence fetus development and outcomes during infancy not limited to the immune system and the response to infections, but involving also brain functional domains.

According to other elaborations, antibiotic administration seems related to behavioral disorders, later in life, because of the drastic impact on the microbial community. Accordingly, the present report highlights the interactions of the microbiome-gut-brain axis and underlines the importance of maintaining the healthy commensal gut microbiota to ensure a physiological neurodevelopment. But many details and processes still need to be clarified, and future trials could hopefully investigate this relation as a primary outcome.

Neurodevelopment: the impact of nutrition and inflammation during early to middle childhood in low-resource settings

John CC[1], Black MM[2–4], Nelson III CA[5–7]

[1]Ryan White Center for Pediatric Infectious Disease and Global Health, Indiana University School of Medicine, Indianapolis, IN, USA; [2]Departments of Pediatrics and [3]Department of Epidemiology, University of Maryland School of Medicine, Baltimore, MD, USA; [4]RTI International, Research Triangle Park, NC; [5]Laboratories of Cognitive Neuroscience, Boston Children's Hospital, Boston, MA, USA; [6]Department of Pediatrics, Harvard Medical School, Boston, MA, USA; [7]Department of Human Development, Harvard Graduate School of Education, Cambridge, MA, USA

Pediatrics 2017;139(suppl 1):S59–S71

This article will be commented together with the next one.

Assessment of neurodevelopment, nutrition, and inflammation from fetal life to adolescence in low-resource settings

Suchdev PS[1, 2], Boivin MJ[3, 4], Forsyth BW[5], Georgieff MK[6, 7], Guerrant RL[8], Nelson III CA[9–11]

[1]Departments of Pediatrics and [2]Global Health, Emory University, Atlanta, GA, USA; [3]Departments of Psychiatry and [4]Neurology and Ophthalmology, Michigan State University, East Lansing, MI, USA; [5]Department of Pediatrics, Yale University, New Haven, CT, USA; [6]Departments of Pediatrics and [7]Child Psychology, University of Minnesota School of Medicine, Minneapolis, MN, USA; [8]Center for Global Health, Department of Medicine, University of Virginia School of Medicine, Charlottesville, VA, USA; [9]Laboratories of Cognitive Neuroscience, Boston Children's Hospital, Boston, MA, USA; [10]Department of Pediatrics, Harvard Medical School, Boston MA, USA; [11]Harvard Graduate School of Education, Cambridge, MA, USA

Pediatrics 2017;139(suppl 1):S23–S37

Reviews: These 2 review articles provide an overview of key definitions, tools, and applications relevant to the assessment of neurodevelopment, nutrition, inflammation, and infection and identify critical research gaps and priorities.

The critical periods that have been identified are respectively, from fetal life to adolescence and during early to middle childhood in low-resource settings (LRS).

Comments Children in LRS might be exposed to negative experiences that influence gene expression, which may play a role on the neurodevelopment and also on the behavioral development. For these reasons, children in LRS might be at risk for falling off a normal growth trajectory.

As for the assessment of nutrition, an optimal nutritional status is essential to ensure a normal neurodevelopment. Malnutrition, considered as undernutrition, deficiencies in micronutrients, and overweight/obesity, has been identified as risk factors to the developing brain.

Another aspect considered in these reports is the role of inflammation on brain growth and function. The available evidence suggests that fetal exposure to maternal infection and inflammation may have a profound effect on neurodevelopment during childhood.

The interactions between inflammation and nutrition are complex and bidirectional. Microbiome and environmental conditions represent 2 recent areas of interest that may have an interactive effect in later life.

Newer and original studies are needed to clarify the direct effects of inflammation and nutrition on neurodevelopment and, in particular, interventions that can favorably impact these relationships.

Association between maternal nutritional status in pregnancy and offspring cognitive function during childhood and adolescence: a systematic review

Veena SR[1], Gale CR[2, 3], Krishnaveni GV[1], Kehoe SH[2], Srinivasan K[4], Fall CHD[2]

[1]Epidemiology Research Unit, CSI Holdsworth Memorial Hospital, Mysore, India; [2]MRC Lifecourse Epidemiology Unit, University of Southampton, Southampton, UK; [3]Department of Psychology, Centre for Cognitive Ageing and Cognitive Epidemiology, University of Edinburgh, Edinburgh, UK; [4]St. John's Research Institute, St. John's National Academy of Health Sciences, Bangalore, India

BMC Pregnancy Childbirth 2016;16:220

Background: During gestation, food habits and consequently nutritional status of women are crucial for the normal brain growth of their children.

Methods: The authors have focused their attention on BMI, height and weight; status or intake of selected single micronutrients (vitamins D, B1, B6, B12 and folate, and iron), and dietary intake of macronutrients (carbohydrate, protein, and fat) in pregnant women. From the database search, any measure of neurocognitive outcomes in children up to 18 years of age, were examined. They observed clinical trials, observational studies from retrieved literature and identified 16,143 articles published in English from January 1960 to October 2014, excluding case reports and animal studies.

Results: Based on inclusion criteria, 38 articles were selected. The investigators obtained controversial results. Maternal obesity and vitamin D deficiency seem to be associated with lower neurocognitive performance of their children. Most studies found no association between maternal vitamin B12 and iron status and offspring cognitive function.

Two trials, one of maternal carbohydrate/protein supplementation and the other of folic acid supplementation showed no effects on the children's neurocognitive outcomes. Since positive findings were mainly in observational studies, residual confounding limits conclusions.

Conclusions: There is inconclusive evidence to confirm or refute the association of maternal nutritional status (BMI, single micronutrient or macronutrient intakes) with offspring cognitive function.

Comments The major limitation in the present knowledge on this topic is represented by the very limited number of studies and/or observations from the poorer developing countries. Indeed, mothers coming from these settings should reasonably be more exposed to nutritional deficiencies, and yet more advantaged by specific supplementations. It is likely the only way to convincingly show the potential of a given nutrient on brain functional development.

Maternal dietary patterns during pregnancy and intelligence quotients in the offspring at 8 years of age: findings from the ALSPAC cohort

Freitas Vilela AA[1], Pearson RM[2], Emmett P[2], Heron J[2], Smith AD[2], Emond A[2], Hibbeln JR[3], Castro MBT[1], Kac G[1]

[1]Nutritional Epidemiology Observatory, Department of Social and Applied Nutrition, Institute of Nutrition Josué de Castro, Rio de Janeiro Federal University, Rio de Janeiro, Brazil; [2]School of Social and Community Medicine, University of Bristol, Bristol, UK; [3]Section of Nutritional Neurosciences, Laboratory of Membrane Biology and Biophysics, National Institute on Alcohol Abuse and Alcoholism, National Institutes of Health, Bethesda, MD, USA

Matern Child Nutr 2018;14:e12431

Background: Maternal nutritional status during gestation has been identified as an important aspect of the developing brain of offspring.
Children of women who have an adequate dietary intake during pregnancy show better cognitive outcomes compared to children of women who follow an unbalanced diet.
Methods: The aim of the present study was to examine the links between maternal dietary patterns during pregnancy and IQ of their children at 8 years of age, assessed using the Wechsler Intelligence Scale for Children.
Results: Maternal food habits were obtained by cluster analysis during pregnancy; 47 food items were used and accordingly mothers classified into 3 best described clusters: "fruit and vegetables," "meat and potatoes," and "white bread and coffee." Pregnant women who were classified in the fruit and vegetables cluster had offspring with higher average IQ compared to the other 2 groups.
Conclusions: Maternal diet in pregnancy may promote an optimal neurodevelopment in offspring when following a diet rich in fruit and vegetables.

Comments   In previous publications, the authors concluded that current evidence about the role of BMI, single micronutrient or macronutrient intakes of pregnant women on offspring cognitive function is inconclusive.

In the second study, the results showed that children of women in "fruit and vegetables" cluster had the highest mean verbal, performance, and full-scale IQ scores at 8 years of age compared to children with mothers classified in the others clusters, and children of women in "white bread and coffee" had the lowest average scores. This study, whose observations are highly interesting like other previously published from the same group, presents some limitations, as well as, loss to follow-up of subjects from the original sample, missing data, and underestimation or overestimation of dietary intake through the food frequency questionnaire.

Therefore, many unclear aspects may still confound the evidence. The general common-sense recommendation is still working, that is, during gestation, maternal food habits should be optimal to ensure a normal neurodevelopment in the offspring. Newer and original studies are needed, in particular in less well-nourished populations, to examine these associations.

From neuro-pigments to neural efficiency: the relationship between retinal carotenoids and behavioral and neuroelectric indices of cognitive control in *childhood*

Walk AM[1], Khan NA[1, 2], Barnett SM[3], Raine LB[4], Kramer AF[4, 5], Cohen NJ[5, 6], Moulton CJ[7], Renzi-Hammond LM[8], Hammond BR[8]; Hillman CH[4, 9]

[1]Department of Kinesiology and Community Health, University of Illinois, USA; [2]Division of Nutritional Sciences, University of Illinois, USA; [3]Department of Food Science, Washington State University, USA; [4]Department of Psychology, Northeastern University, USA; [5]Beckman Institute of Science and Technology, University of Illinois, USA; [6]Department of Psychology University of Illinois, USA; [7]Abbott Nutrition, USA; [8]Behavioral and Brain Sciences, University of Georgia, USA; [9]Department of Health Science, Northeastern University, USA

Int J Psychophysiol 2017;118:1–8

Background: Lutein and zeaxanthin are 2 carotenoids present in nature and in the human diet, highly concentrated as macular pigments in the foveal retina of primates. Lutein, in particular, is known to accumulate across all cortices and brain membranes. Recent studies have focused the attention on the possible function of lutein on maintaining the cognitive abilities in older adults.

Few investigations have examined the relationship between lutein and cognition in living children. The present study is the first to explore lutein in relation to any brain-based measure of cognition in preadolescent children.

Methods: By 2 testing sessions, authors examined participants' cognitive performance (response accuracy and reaction time). Children completed Macular Pigment Optical Density assessment, a retinal measure that is sensitive to cognitive measures, and an educational achievement test. Furthermore, an electroencephalogram was recorded.

Results: Results presented suggest that lutein is involved in cognitive control. Children with higher Macular Pigment Optical Density values show better neural efficiency but with neural markers of lower cognitive load.

Conclusions: The potential positive function of lutein to cognitive performance should be investigated during the lifespan to extend present findings and improve cognition in childhood.

Comments Welcome to the entry into the arena of *food for thought*, another micronutrient, lutein, is still under discussion to extract a functional role on brain in early life. Whatever the results and the role, we expect harmonization of studies before reaching non-conclusive evidence for other most popular compounds.

Overall Summary

The indications that can be drawn from the presented papers may be summarized in few points:

1   When studying a nutrient, harmonization among studies (and not just in the field of effects on cognition) is mandatory, not to waste money with heterogeneous study designs and allowing for comparisons between results, in order to reach firm conclusions.

2   Newer and most solid neurodevelopmental tests are needed, considering different ages and cultural background, and not contaminated by the use in clinical practice of scales born to score the mental handicap, since we need to study effects within the normal range of intellectual achievement.

3   While most controversial studies probably arise from the typical western models, where all conditions are more favorable in general, and differences of effects are blunted, future studies should

consider trials in developing and transition countries, where effects on developmental achievement could have more striking effects.

If studies and research in the field do not evolve further, it is hard that in the next years we could evolve from the present status, where many single studies suggest mild effects of intervention (if any) and systematic reviews and metanalyses end with the frustrating sentence on "more well-designed studies are needed."

Koletzko B, Shamir R, Turck D, Phillip M (eds): Nutrition and Growth: Yearbook 2018.
World Rev Nutr Diet. Basel, Karger, 2018, vol 117, pp 84–110 (DOI: 10.1159/000484501)

Nutrition and Growth in Chronic Disease

Corina Hartman[1] · Raanan Shamir[2,3]

[1]Pediatric Gastroenterolgy and Nutrition Unit, Lady Davis Carmel Medical Center, Haifa, [2]Institute of Gastroenterology, Nutrition and Liver Diseases, Schneider Children's Medical Center of Israel, Clalit Health Services, Petach Tikva, and [3]Sackler Faculty of Medicine, Tel Aviv University, Tel Aviv, Israel

Environmental, behavioral (nutrition and physical activity), and disease-related factors can prevent attainment of full genetic potential for growth. Undernutrition is most often the cause of growth faltering and poor skeletal development. Disease-related factors, such as malabsorption, inflammation, and immobility also have profound effects. These effects are illustrated in selected abstracts in this chapter discussing diseases such as inflammatory bowel disease (IBD), cystic fibrosis (CF), celiac disease (CD), and children with food allergies. This overview of health and disease effects on growth and skeletal development provides insights into the plasticity of human growth and its sensitivity to the overall health or diseases.

Key articles reviewed for this chapter

Inflammatory Bowel Disease

Growth improvement with adalimumab treatment in children with moderately to severely active Crohn's disease

Walters TD, Faubion WA, Griffiths AM, Baldassano RN, Escher J, Ruemmele FM, Hyams JS, Lazar A, Eichner S, Huang B, Li Y, Thakkar RB

Inflamm Bowel Dis 2017;23:967–975

Changes in hepcidin and hemoglobin after anti-TNF-alpha therapy in children and adolescents with Crohn's disease

Atkinson MA, Leonard MB, Herskovitz R, Baldassano RN, Denburg MR

J Pediatr Gastroenterol Nutr 2017, Epub ahead of print

Correction of iron deficiency anemia with intravenous iron sucrose in children with inflammatory bowel disease

Danko I, Weidkamp M

J Pediatr Gastroenterol Nutr 2016;63:e107–e111

Cystic Fibrosis

Effects of diagnosis by newborn screening for cystic fibrosis on weight and length in the first year of life

Leung DH, Heltshe SL, Borowitz D, Gelfond D, Kloster M, Heubi JE, Stalvey M, Ramsey BW; for the Baby Observational and Nutrition Study (BONUS) Investigators of the Cystic Fibrosis Foundation Therapeutics Development Network

JAMA Pediatr 2017;171:546–554

Differences in outcomes between early and late diagnosis of cystic fibrosis in the newborn screening era

Coffey MJ, Whitaker V, Gentin N, Junek R, Shalhoub C, Nightingale S, Hilton J, Wiley V, Wilcken B, Gaskin KJ, Ooi CY

J Pediatr 2017;181:137–145.e1

Differences between WHO and CDC early growth measurements in the assessment of cystic fibrosis clinical outcomes

Usatin D, Yen EH, McDonald C, Asfour F, Pohl J, Robson J

J Cyst Fibros 2017;16:503–509

Macronutrient intake in preschoolers with cystic fibrosis and the relationship between macronutrients and growth

Filigno SS, Robson SM, Szczesniak RD, Chamberlin LA, Baker MA, Sullivan SM, Kroner J, Powers SW

J Cyst Fibros 2017;16:519–524

Celiac Disease

Celiac disease is associated with reduced bone mineral density and increased FRAX scores in the US national health and nutrition examination survey

Kamycheva E, Goto T, Camargo CA Jr

Osteoporosis Int 2017;28:781–790

Reduced bone mineral density in children with screening-detected celiac disease

Björck S, Brundin C, Karlsson M, Agardh D

J Pediatr Gastroenterol Nutr 2017;65:526–532

At-risk screened children with celiac disease are comparable in disease severity and dietary adherence to those found because of clinical suspicion: a large cohort study

Kivelä L, Kaukinen K, Huhtala H, Lähdeaho ML, Mäki M, Kurppa K

J Pediatr 2017;183:115–121.e2

Early growth in children with celiac disease: a cohort study

Kahrs CR, Magnus MC, Stigum H, Lundin KEA, Størdal K

Arch Dis Child 2017;102:1037–1043

Food Allergy

The impact of the elimination diet on growth and nutrient intake in children with food protein induced gastrointestinal allergies

Meyer R, De Koker C, Dziubak R, Godwin H, Dominguez-Ortega G, Chebar Lozinsky A, Skrapac AK, Gholmie Y, Reeve K, Shah N

Clin Transl Allergy 2016;6:25

Iodine status and growth in 0- to 2-year-old infants with cow's milk protein allergy

Thomassen RA, Kvammen JA, Eskerud MB, Júlíusson PB, Henriksen C, Rugtveit J

J Pediatr Gastroenterol Nutr 2017;64:806–811

Attention Deficit/Hyperactivity Disorder

Association of stimulant medication use with bone mass in children and adolescents with attention-deficit/hyperactivity disorder

Feuer AJ, Thai A, Demmer RT, Vogiatzi M

JAMA Pediatr 2016;170:e162804

Growth improvement with adalimumab treatment in children with moderately to severely active Crohn's disease

Walters TD[1], Faubion WA[2], Griffiths AM[1], Baldassano RN[3], Escher J[4], Ruemmele FM[5], Hyams JS[6], Lazar A[7], Eichner S[8], Huang B[8], Li Y[8], Thakkar RB[8]

[1]Department of Gastroenterology, Hepatology and Nutrition, The Hospital for Sick Children, Toronto, Ontario, Canada; [2]Department of Gastroenterology and Hepatology, Mayo Clinic, Rochester, MN, USA; [3]Department of Pediatrics, Children's Hospital of Philadelphia, Philadelphia, PA, USA; [4]Department of Pediatric Gastroenterology, Erasmus MC-Sophia Children's Hospital, Rotterdam, The Netherlands; [5]Department of Pediatrics, Pediatric Gastroenterology, Universite Sorbonne Paris-Cite, Hospital Necker-Enfants Malades, Paris, France; [6]Division of Digestive Diseases, Hepatology and Nutrition, Connecticut Children's Medical Center, Hartford, CT, USA; [7]AbbVie Deutschland GmbH & Co. KG, Ludwigshafen, Germany; [8]AbbVie Inc., North Chicago, IL, USA

Inflamm Bowel Dis 2017;23:967–975

Background: The IMAgINE 1 trial investigated the efficacy and safety of adalimumab (ADA), a fully human monoclonal antibody against tumor necrosis factor (TNF)-α, for induction and maintenance of remission in children with moderately to severely active Crohn's disease (CrD). The present study reported the effect of ADA on height velocity in pediatric patients with impaired baseline linear growth, participants in the IMAgINE 1 trial.

Methods: IMAgINE 1 was a 52-week, phase 3, multicenter, randomized, double-blind trial that assessed the efficacy and safety of 2 induction doses (160/80 vs. 80/40 mg) and 2 maintenance dose regimens (40 vs. 20 mg) of ADA in 6- to 17-year-old patients with moderately to severely active CrD. The children reported in this analysis were a subset of patients from the IMAgINE 1 trial, considered to have growth potential, that is, females with a bone age <13 years and males with a bone age <14 years.

Results: The IMAgINE 1 trial enrolled 100 patients, majority of whom (73/100, 73%) had linear growth impairment at baseline (height velocity z-score <−1.0). During the 52 weeks of ADA therapy, linear growth normalized in patients who initially had significant impairment at baseline. The median height velocity z-score improved from -3.25 at baseline to −0.34 by 26 weeks, and further improved to +0.21 by 52 weeks. By week 26 and also at week 52, there was no significant difference in linear growth rate between the group with initial impairment compared with those with normal linear growth at baseline.

Patients who received high-dose ADA had greater median height velocity z-scores compared with patients who received low-dose ADA at both 26 and 52 weeks. The median height velocity z-score at 52 weeks was +0.67 for the high-dose and −0.42 for the low-dose ADA group.

Patients receiving ADA without dose escalation had greater median height velocity z-scores compared with patients who required dose escalation to weekly ADA. The median height velocity at 52 weeks was +1.71 in patients without dose escalation and −1.36 in patients whose dose escalated ($p < 0.007$). Patients with baseline growth impairment, who were responders to ADA induction therapy, achieved a significant growth improvement by week 26 but nonsignificant although numerical different at week 52 compared with non-responders at week 4. The median height velocity z-score at 26 weeks was +0.09 vs. −2.92, $p = 0.023$ and +0.68 vs. −1.78, $p = 0.160$ at 52 weeks, in responders vs. non-responders. Week 4 response status was a significant predictor of linear growth normalization at week 26 (OR 9.28 [95% CI 1.39–62.10]; $p < 0.022$). ADA trough levels at week 4 after induction therapy were also a significant predictor of growth normalization (OR 1.13 [95% CI 1.01–1.27]; $p <$ 0.033). ROC curve analysis suggested that an ADA trough concentration of 10.9 mg/mL was the best cutoff for growth normalization in this patient population (area under the ROC curve, 0.605). At week 52, male patients were significantly more likely to exhibit normalization in height velocity than female patients (OR 4.04 [95% CI 1.12–14.50]; $p < 0.032$).

Patients treated with ADA with linear growth impairment at baseline who achieved and maintained durable remission throughout the study (defined by pediatric Crohn's disease activity index [PCDAI] <10 at >80% of visits after week 4) were significantly more likely to exhibit a normal growth rate at week 52 than patients without durable remission ($p < 0.023$). Disease severity and corticosteroids use prior to trial had no impact on growth velocity during ADA treatment.

Conclusion: ADA therapy significantly improved linear growth rate in pediatric patients with baseline growth retardation enrolled in the IMAgINE 1 trial. Restoration of normal growth was significantly associated with clinical remission and was especially profound in week 4 responders and in patients with higher ADA blood levels.

Comments   CrD is a progressive inflammatory disorder of the gastrointestinal tract. About 15% to 25% of IBD cases occur in children and adolescents. Growth, nutritional problems, and delayed pubertal development are common complications in pediatric CrD. Restoration of linear growth and achievement of the full growth potential are as important as maintaining disease remission and quality of life. Growth failure in children with CrD is multifactorial and involves chronic inflammation, undernutrition, corticosteroid therapy, and insulin-like growth factor-1 (IGF-1) growth hormone axis dysfunction [1]. Among the therapeutic strategies used in children and adolescents with CrD, some were also shown to improve growth, that is, nutritional interventions such as exclusive enteral nutrition used for induction of remission, surgery in patients with limited disease, and anti-TNF-α treatment. Data from clinical trials have shown that anti TNF-α therapy can improve height velocity in children with CrD. Furthermore, early treatment with anti TNF-α (less than 3 months after diagnosis) starting before or in early puberty leads to greater improvement in height and height velocity with Infliximab (IFX; a chimeric anti-TNF-α antibody) [2].

ADA, a fully human monoclonal antibody, is approved for use in children aged 6–17 years with moderately to severely active CrD (United States and Europe). The results of this study showed that ADA was an effective treatment for inducing and maintaining clinical response and remission in children, who had failed conventional therapies or previous anti TNF-α therapy. Children with moderately to severely active CrD who completed the IMAgINE 1 trial through week 52 and who had responded to treatment entered the open-label extension IMAgINE 2 study.

Children with no linear growth impairment at baseline maintained their growth velocity over time. In patients with growth retardation at baseline, linear growth normalized during the 52 weeks of ADA therapy. Indeed, by week 26, there was no significant difference in linear growth rate between the groups with initial growth impairment compared with those with normal linear growth at baseline. This growth rate was maintained at week 52. The growth velocity rate was higher in patients on high-dose ADA, in patients who were responders to ADA induction therapy at 4 weeks and ADA naïve patients. ADA trough levels at week 4 after induction therapy were a significant predictor of growth normalization and ADA trough concentration of 10.9 mg/mL was the best cutoff for growth normalization in this patient population. Male patients were significantly more likely to exhibit normalization in height velocity than female patients at 52 weeks. Growth velocity during ADA treatment was not influenced by disease severity but patients with linear growth impairment who achieved and maintained durable remission throughout the study were significantly more likely to exhibit a normal growth rate at week 52 than patients without durable remission.

It can be concluded that full growth potential in children and adolescents with CrD is achievable today in the era of biologic therapy. Timely use of biologic therapy, keeping the disease under control, and maintaining good nutritional status may improve the chances of children and adolescents with significant growth retardation to achieve their growth potential and predicted height as adults.

Changes in hepcidin and hemoglobin after anti-TNF-alpha therapy in children and adolescents with Crohn's disease

Atkinson MA[1], Leonard MB[2], Herskovitz R[3], Baldassano RN[4], Denburg MR[3]

[1]Department of Pediatrics, Division of Pediatric Nephrology, Johns Hopkins University School of Medicine, Baltimore, MD, USA; [2]Departments of Pediatrics and Medicine, Division of Nephrology, Stanford University School of Medicine, Stanford, CA, USA; [3]Departments of Pediatrics and Epidemiology, The Children's Hospital of Philadelphia, Perelman School of Medicine at the University of Pennsylvania, Philadelphia, PA; USA; [4]Department of Pediatrics, Division of Gastroenterology, Hepatology and Nutrition, The Children's Hospital of Philadelphia Perelman School of Medicine of the University of Pennsylvania, Philadelphia, PA, USA

J Pediatr Gastroenterol Nutr 2017, Epub ahead of print

Background: Anemia is the most common nutritional deficiency in patients with IBD. The pathophysiology of anemia involves poor intake but also defective absorption, gastrointestinal blood loss, and chronic inflammation. The main key mediator of anemia of chronic inflammation is the iron-regulatory protein, hepcidin. The present study investigated prospectively, the serum hepcidin levels in children and adolescents with CrD at baseline and 10 weeks after anti-TNF-therapy.

Methods: Serum hepcidin-25 and hemoglobin (Hb) were measured in 40 children and adolescents with CrD at baseline and 10 weeks after initiation of anti-TNF therapy. Measures of disease activity, inflammatory markers, and cytokines were obtained in all subjects. Anemia was defined by World Health Organization (WHO) criteria (Hb <11.5 g/dL in children aged 2–11 years, Hb <12 g/dL in females aged >12 years, Hb <13 g/dL in males 12–18 years, and <13.5 g/dL in males >18 years).

Results: The mean Hb was 10.6 ± 1.2 g/dL and 95% of subjects were anemic at baseline. Only serum C-reactive protein (CRP) was positively correlated with hepcidin concentrations at baseline ($r = 0.34$, $p = 0.03$). After anti-TNF therapy, at 10 weeks, median (interquartile range [IQR]) hepcidin concentrations decreased significantly (27.9 [16.2–52.9] vs. 23.2 [11.1–37.7] ng/mL, $p = 0.01$). Mean $\pm$ SD Hb also increased significantly (10.6 $\pm$ 1.2 to 10.9 $\pm$ 1.1 g/dL, $p = 0.02$), and the increase was sustained at 12 months, although 90% of participants continued to meet anemia criteria at 10 weeks. Disease activity and markers of inflammation also decreased and albumin levels increased. Higher TNF-α, interleukin (IL)-6, ESR, and CRP were associated with higher hepcidin concentrations ($p = 0.04$, $p = 0.03$, $p = 0.003$, and $p < 0.001$, respectively). Increased levels of disease activity, as evaluated by PCDAI were also associated with higher hepcidin.

Conclusions: In children with CrD, anti-TNF therapy was associated with decreased levels of hepcidin and increased Hb 10 weeks after induction, suggesting that the anti-inflammatory actions of TNF-α blockade may extend to suppression of the specific stimuli for hepcidin production. This further supports a link between hepcidin, abnormal iron homeostasis, inflammatory cytokines, and CrD activity. Improvement in anemia may be a secondary benefit for children who receive this therapy.

Comments Anemia is the most common nutritional complication of IBD. The prevalence of anemia is reported to be as high as 77% in children and 42% in adolescents, compared to 40% in adults [3]. Anemia is associated with impaired growth, poor quality of life due to increased fatigue, and decrease in cognitive function. The etiology of anemia in IBD is multifactorial due in part to inflammation, chronic blood loss, and poor iron/micronutrient intake. Iron supplementation by enteral and/ or intravenous (IV) route is the mainstay of therapy for iron deficiency anemia but inflammation-mediated impaired iron trafficking often results in resistance to these treatments. There is now consensus that anemia of chronic inflammation is at large a consequence of altered iron metabolism facilitated by inflammatory mediators. Immune mediators, such as IL-6 and possibly other cytokines involved in host defense, lead to hepcidin-induced hypoferremia, resulting in iron sequestration within the reticuloendothelial system and decreased iron availability for erythropoiesis [4]. Hepcidin is the principal regulator of iron homeostasis, including dietary iron absorption, iron recycling by macrophages, and the release of iron from hepatic stores. Hepcidin expression is induced by circulating iron and tissue iron stores, as well as inflammatory cytokines and suppressed by hypoxia, iron deficiency, and ineffective erythropoiesis. Hepcidin binding to its receptor causes internalization and degradation of ferroportin (the sole iron exporter), resulting in down-regulation of dietary iron absorption by intestinal enterocytes and inhibition of stored iron release from reticuloendothelial cells, preventing the utilization of absorbed or stored iron for erythropoiesis in the bone marrow.

Therapeutic monoclonal antibodies against IL-6 receptor (tocilizumab), IL-6 (siltuximab), and TNFα (golimumab or IFX) were shown to decrease hepcidin and improve anemia [5].

Prior studies have shown that compared to healthy controls, serum levels of hepcidin were elevated in adults with CrD and were positively correlated with disease activity and serum concentrations CRP and IL-6 and negatively correlated with Hb levels [6]. The decrease in hepcidin levels, in this study, associated with a concurrent marked decrease in cytokines, inflammatory markers, and CrD activity, suggests that the anti-inflammatory actions of TNF-α blockade may extend to the suppression of specific stimuli for hepcidin production, in addition to a small increase in Hb. These findings suggest that stimuli for hepcidin transcription are relieved after anti-TNF induction, supporting a link between hepcidin, abnormal iron homeostasis, inflammatory cytokines, and CrD activity. Although treatment of the underlying disease remains at the center of therapy for inflammatory diseases, recent advances in molecular understanding of the hepcidin-ferroportin axis are stimulating the development of new targeted therapies.

Correction of iron deficiency anemia with intravenous iron sucrose in children with inflammatory bowel disease

Danko I, Weidkamp M

Department of Pediatrics, Division of Gastroenterology, Hepatology and Nutrition, University of Wisconsin, School of Medicine and Public Health, Madison, WI, USA

J Pediatr Gastroenterol Nutr 2016;63:e107–e111

Aims: Iron deficiency anemia (IDA) is common in children with IBD. Oral iron supplementation has serious limitations including poor adherence, adverse effects, and iron malabsorption related to bowel inflammation. The objective of this study was to evaluate the feasibility and efficacy of periodic IV iron treatments for correction of IDA in children with IBD.

Methods: This prospective study was conducted in 24 children with IBD treated with IFX, 21/24 with CrD. Participants received 3 mg/kg (maximum 200 mg) IV iron sucrose (IS) after each IFX treatments if they were iron deficient according to the following criteria:
1 Ferritin <30 ng/mL or transferrin saturation (TSAT) <20% with normal CRP, or
2 Ferritin <100 ng/mL and TSAT <20% with elevated CRP.
They continued to receive IV IS with each IFX treatment until 2 consecutive laboratories showed no evidence of iron deficiency. Disease activity (PCDAI or pediatric ulcerative colitis index), hematology, and iron indices obtained during the study were compared with historical data from the same patients.

Results: The participants received a total of 138 IS infusions. The mean (±SD) number of infusions was 5.6 (±3.7) with a range of 2–18 per individual patient. The frequency of IS infusions ranged from 0.5 to 2.7 bimonthly. The mean ferritin (±SE) rose from 21.9 (±3.2) to 48.8 (±6.3) ng/mL ($p = 0.0004$), TSAT (±SE) from 13.2 (±1.8) to 23.6 (±2.6)%, ($p = 0.0009$), and Hb (±SE) from 11.4 (±0.3) to 12.7 (±0.3) g/dL, ($p = 0.006$). The proportion of patients with normal mean ferritin, TSAT, and Hb rose from 33 to 75% ($p = 0.002$), 21–63% ($p = 0.006$), and 25–79% ($p = 0.0002$), respectively. One patient with ulcerative colitis (pancolitis) was a nonresponder and 6 other patients, 4 with CrD and 2 with ulcerative colitis were relatively poor responders with an increase in mean Hb of <0.5 g/dL. All poor responders had a normal mean post-IS CRP, and, except 2 patients all had mean disease activity <10. No adverse reactions were reported.

Conclusions: The study shows that incorporation of IV IS into routine management of IDA in children with IBD is feasible, safe, and effective. This approach overcomes the 2 major obstacles that impede successful management of IDA in these patients, namely non-adherence with oral iron supplements and poor iron absorption associated with chronic inflammation.

Comments The anemia of patients with IBD is at many times the result of a combination of dysregulated iron trafficking due to chronic inflammation and iron deficiency. The decision to whether supplemental iron is needed in a patient with IBD and anemia should be preceded by careful evaluation of iron status, including information on Hb, mean corpuscular volume, serum ferritin, and TSAT. In addition, inflammatory markers such as CRP must be taken into consideration. Interpretation of iron stores based on serum ferritin may be misleading since ferritin, as an acute-phase reactant, may be normal or elevated even in the presence of iron deficiency. For this reason, ferritin levels, up to 100 µg/L, may still be consistent with iron deficiency, in the presence of elevated inflammatory markers.

The treatment with oral iron has significant limitations in IBD, being less efficient than the IV route. In addition, unabsorbed iron may harm intestinal mucosa and worsen IBD symptoms by aggravating intestinal inflammation. Oral iron supplementation may also affect microbiota and increases fecal calprotectin [6]. Taking into account these possible effects, the recently published European Crohn's and Colitis Organisation (ECCO) guidelines state that the IV route should be preferred in the patients with IBD [7]. IV preparations have the advantage of bypassing intestinal absorption and compliance problems as iron replacement can be achieved with few doses of the newer high-dose preparations.

There are a number of different IV iron formulations: high and low molecular weight iron dextran, IS, ferric gluconate, ferric carboxymaltose and ferumoxytol. As IV iron preparations have different physicochemical properties, the administration requires different dosages: more frequent lower individual doses are needed for IS or gluconate, whereas more stable preparations (e.g., iron dextran or ferric carboxymaltose) can be given as large single IV doses [8]. Concerns regarding the safety of IV iron preparations refer particularly to high molecular weight dextran formulations, which have an increased risk of anaphylaxis resulting from anti-dextran antibodies. Newer IV iron drugs such as IS and ferric carboxymaltose have been studied in few children with IBD and appear to have good safety profiles, high efficacy, and improved compliance as fewer IV doses are needed to correct iron deficiency (carboxymaltose) [9]. This study is the first prospective study that reported the efficacy of an IV iron preparation in the treatment of IDA in children with IBD. Further studies using the new high-dose iron preparations are awaited.

Cystic Fibrosis

Effects of diagnosis by newborn screening for cystic fibrosis on weight and length in the first year of life

Leung DH[1], Heltshe SL[2, 3], Borowitz D[4, 5], Gelfond D[6], Kloster M[2], Heubi JE[7, 8], Stalvey M[9], Ramsey BW[2, 3]; for the Baby Observational and Nutrition Study (BONUS) Investigators of the Cystic Fibrosis Foundation Therapeutics Development Network

[1]Division of Gastroenterology, Hepatology, and Nutrition, Department of Pediatrics, Baylor College of Medicine, Houston, TX, USA; [2]Cystic Fibrosis Foundation Therapeutics Development Network Coordinating Center, Seattle Children's Research Institute, Seattle, WA, USA; [3]Division of Pulmonary and Sleep Medicine, Department of Pediatrics, University of Washington, Seattle, WA, USA; [4]Department of Pediatrics, University of Buffalo, Buffalo, NY, USA; [5]Cystic Fibrosis Foundation, Bethesda, MD, USA; [6]Division of Gastroenterology/Nutrition, Department of Pediatrics, University of Rochester, Rochester, NY, USA; [7]Division of Gastroenterology and Nutrition, Cincinnati Children's Hospital Medical Center, Cincinnati, OH, USA; [8]Department of Pediatrics, University of Cincinnati College of Medicine, Cincinnati, OH, USA; [9]Department of Pediatrics, University of Alabama at Birmingham, Birmingham, AL, USA

JAMA Pediatr 2017;171:546–554

Aims: To examine the growth (weight gain and linear growth) status in the first year of life in infants with CF diagnosed by newborn screening (NBS) for CF. Furthermore, the study explored concurrent nutritional, metabolic, respiratory, infectious, and inflammatory characteristics associated with early CF anthropometric measurements.

Methods: The study evaluated infants prospectively enrolled in the Baby Observational and Nutrition Study (BONUS), a prospective multicenter study of infants with CF. Study visits coincided with guideline-recommended CF clinic visits (monthly until 6 months and at 8, 10, and 12 months of age) and included anthropometry, diet records, fecal elastase levels, respiratory tract cultures, and chest radiography (according to CF Foundation care guidelines). Clinical data, dietary intake, hematology, biochemistry, and serum vitamin levels (A, D, and E) were collected at enrollment and at 6 and 12 months.

Results: The BONUS cohort consisted of 231 infants with CF, 215 (93.1%) completed follow-up through 12 months of age.

Weight: Birth weights of BONUS infants were statistically lower than those of WHO healthy newborns (mean z-score, –0.15; 95% CI –0.27 to –0.04), with a median birth weight of 3.2 (range 2.5–4.4) kg. By 12 months of age, BONUS infants demonstrated increased weight gain, and weight for age was not different from that of WHO healthy infants (mean z-score, –0.04; 95% CI –0.17 to 0.09) and better than the 1994–1995 CF birth cohort.

Length: Birth lengths of BONUS infants were higher than those of WHO healthy newborns (mean z-score, 0.44; 95% CI 0.26–0.62), with a median birth length of 50.8 (range 40.1–57.3) cm. However, length for age in BONUS infants was lower than that in WHO healthy infants at 3, 6, and 12 months of age (12-month mean z-score, –0.56; 95% CI –0.70 to –0.42). Length was improved compared with the historic cohort at 6 months (z-score increase, 1.06; 95% CI 0.82–1.30) and at 12 months (z score increase, 0.63; 95% CI 0.41–0.86).

Feeding: The median caloric intake in the first year was 107 kcal/kg/day (range 86–133 kcal/kg/day).

Exclusively breastfed infants weighed more than formula-fed infants or those fed a combination at 3 months of age (mean z-score difference, 0.54; 95% CI 0.22–0.87) but not at 6 or 12 months. Feeding type was not associated with infant length at any time point.

Using cumulative anthropometrics through the first year, participants were categorized into low-weight and low-length groups. Among the 222 BONUS infants with follow-up beyond 6 months, 30 (13.6%) had low-weight; 53 (23.9%) low-length; and 24 (10.8%) had both. Low-weight infants consumed significantly more calories than did normal-weight infants at 6 months (153 vs. 101 kcal/kg/day). Low-length infants also consumed significantly more calories (131 vs. 100 kcal/kg/day).

Associations between growth and clinical features: Weight and length z-scores of infants from the BONUS cohort were affected by the class of disease mutations, presence of pancreatic insufficiency (PI), meconium ileus, gender, presence of *Pseudomonas aeruginosa* colonization of respiratory tract and wheezing.

Conclusions: Although z-score for weight for age lagged behind WHO normative values at birth and during the first 6 months of age, BONUS infants' z-score for weight increased to those of WHO healthy infants by 12 months. Correction in weight gain was a striking improvement compared with a 1994–1995 historic cohort, before universal NBS for CF in the United States. In contrast to weight improvement, most infants showed persistent delay in linear growth at 1 year. The study showed that NBS for CF in the United States has likely contributed to the correction of malnutrition and improved suboptimal growth in infants with CF.

Differences in outcomes between early and late diagnosis of cystic fibrosis in the newborn screening era

Coffey MJ[1], Whitaker V[1], Gentin N[1, 2], Junek R[3], Shalhoub C[4], Nightingale S[5, 6], Hilton J[7, 8], Wiley V[3, 9], Wilcken B[3, 9], Gaskin KJ[3, 9], Ooi CY[1, 10]

[1]School of Women's and Children's Health, Faculty of Medicine, University of New South Wales, Sydney, Australia; [2]Department of General Pediatrics, Sydney Children's Hospital Randwick, Sydney, Australia; [3]The Children's Hospital at Westmead, Sydney, Australia; [4]Department of Medical Genetics, Sydney Children's Hospital Randwick, Sydney, Australia; [5]GrowUpWell Priority Research Centre, University of Newcastle, Newcastle, Australia; [6]Department of Gastroenterology, John Hunter Children's Hospital, Newcastle, Australia; [7]University of Newcastle, Newcastle, Australia; [8]Department of Respiratory Medicine, John Hunter Children's Hospital, Newcastle, Australia; [9]The University of Sydney, Sydney, Australia; and [10]Department of Gastroenterology, Sydney Children's Hospital Randwick, Sydney, Australia

J Pediatr 2017;181:137–145.e1

Aims: The study aimed to evaluate and compare the clinical outcomes of patients with CF who had a late diagnosis of CF (LD-CF) despite neonatal screening (NBS), and determined whether their outcomes differ from children diagnosed with CF after a positive NBS and early diagnosis of CF (NBS-CF) during the same time period.

Methods: This retrospective study included all cases with LD-CF identified through the Australian CF Data Registry. As a comparator, each subject with LD-CF was matched 1:2 with patients with NBS-CF for age, sex, exocrine pancreatic status identified through Wisconsin NBS. LD-CF was defined as an individual who fulfilled the criteria for CF and was either (1) NBS negative (LD-NBS-negative) or (2) NBS positive (LD-NBS-positive), but discharged after a sweat test chloride (SC) <60 mmol/L.

Results: A total of 45 LD-CF cases were identified and included along with 90 matched NBS-CF controls. Of the LD-CF cases, 39 were LD-NBS-negative and 6 were LD-NBS positive (2 with a SC <30 mmol/L and 4 with a SC 30–60 mmol/L).

Pancreatic function status was known in 37 of the patients with LD-CF (82%), and of those, 27 (73%) were PI and 10 (27%) were pancreatic sufficient (PS). At the time of diagnosis, 38 patients with LD-CF (84%) and 90 patients with NBS-CF (100%) had manifestations of CF recorded.

The LD-CF cohort presented with significantly more respiratory (66 vs. 4%; $p < 0.0001$), gastrointestinal (24 vs. 6%; $p = 0.005$), and failure to-thrive manifestations (29 vs. 3%; $p < 0.0001$) when compared with NBS-CF controls at the time of diagnosis. The median number of hospital admissions per year for CF-related respiratory illness was significantly higher for patients with LD-CF compared with patients with NBS-CF (0.49 [0.2–1.1] vs. 0.2 [0–0.5] respectively; $p = 0.0004$).

The mean (SD) height z-score was significantly lower for patients with LD-CF compared with NBS-CF (–0.65 [0.22] vs. –0.03 [0.15]; $p = 0.02$). No difference between the LD-CF and NBS-CF cohorts in regard to mean (SD) z-score for weight (–0.48 [0.21] vs. 0.01 [0.14], $p = 9.06$) or body mass index (BMI; –0.11 [0.17] vs. –0.03 [0.12], $p = 0.7$) were evident.

The mean (SD) lung function variables were significantly worse for LD-CF compared with NBS-CF, including forced vital capacity (FVC) (2.1 [0.10] vs. 2.5 L [0.06], $p = 0.003$), forced expiratory volume/1 second (FEV1) (1.7 [0.08] vs. 2.0 L [0.06], $p = 0.003$), and FEV1% (0.88 [0.03] vs. 0.97 [0.02], $p = 0.007$).

Microbiology data showed a significantly higher rate of isolation of *P. aeruginosa* over the duration of follow-up in the LD-CF cohort compared with the NBS-CF cohort (82 vs. 69%, $p = 0.03$).

Conclusions: In this study, children diagnosed lately with CF, most with a false negative NBS result, had significantly worse health at the time of diagnosis, including more respiratory, gastrointestinal, and failure-to-thrive manifestations. Compared with matched controls, children with CF diagnosed earlier by NBS, children with LD-CF had poorer length growth, worse respiratory outcomes including poorer lung function, higher rates of chronic *P. aeruginosa* colonization, and increased frequency of hospitalization for CF-related respiratory illness at follow-up.

Comments   CF is a complex and greatly variable monogenic disease caused by mutations in the CF transmembrane conductance regulator (CFTR) gene on chromosome 7. Airways, pancreas, male genital system, intestine, liver, bone, and kidney are involved. The lack of CFTR or its impaired function causes fat malabsorption and chronic pulmonary infections leading to progressive lung damage. Previously considered lethal in infancy and childhood, the landscape of CF has changed dramatically in the last decade, thanks to the incorporation of new technologies for the diagnosis and treatment of the disease.

Diagnosis based on clinical grounds is usually straightforward in patients with typical manifestations, but occasionally it may be delayed for months. Universal NBS for CF has been implemented in all 50 states in the United States since 2010 and in many countries with a high prevalence of CF around the world [10]. CF NBS programs are based on blood immunoreactive trypsinogen (IRT) measurement in the first days of life followed by, in infants with raised IRT by various combinations of genetic analysis, measurement of pancreatitis-associated protein, and IRT retesting by 1 month of age.

NBS protocols were shown to reduce the therapeutic burden, hospitalization rates, and morbidity associated with CF and are even more significant, especially now in the era of CFTR-targeted therapies for early diagnosis and rescue therapy before irreversible organ damage occurs.

Early diagnosis affords the opportunity to improve long-term outcomes through close monitoring and appropriate interventions beginning before severe nutritional deficits or irreversible airway damage have occurred. As CFTR modulator therapies that treat the basic genetic defect in CF became available across a broad range of ages and CFTR genotypes, initiation of these therapies in infancy holds the promise of changing the disease outcome. However, despite identification of CF in the youngest patients and emphasis on early nutritional supplementation and prompt implementation of pancreatic enzyme replacement therapy (PERT), growth in children with CF continues to lag significantly behind that of healthy children. The good news brought to us by the study by Leung et al. as described on page 92 above, is that, though z-scores for weight for age lagged behind WHO normative values at birth and during the first 6 months of age, BONUS infant z-scores for weight increased compared to those of WHO healthy infants by 12 months. Correction in weight gain represents a striking improvement compared with a 1994–1995 historic cohort, before universal NBS for CF in the United States. Although significant progress was noted in weight gain of infants with CF, a subgroup of infants remained underweight despite increased caloric intake, PERT, and addition of H2 blockers to improve enzyme efficacy. Lung colonization with *P. aeruginosa* and wheezing were associated with the highest risk for low weight or length, even in this very young and relatively healthy population.

In contrast to the weight improvement, linear growth showed persistent delay at 1 year in most BONUS infants. Stunting was not seen in infants with PS. Since pancreatic phenotype is more strongly associated with genotype, patients with PS tend to have milder CFTR mutations (classes IV and V). Although the difference in linear growth between PS and PI children could be attributable to changes in absorption of critical micronutrients, poor growth may ultimately be a consequence of more severe CFTR dysfunction.

An additional finding in the BONUS cohort children was the detection of lower serum IGF-1 levels compared to the values reported in healthy infants. Infants with low length had even lower serum IGF-1 and IGF binding protein 3 levels than the rest of the BONUS cohort. The mechanism behind reduced IGF-1 levels in infants with CF is unknown, but several studies have suggested a direct link between IGF-1 and CFTR dysfunction besides the effect of chronic inflammatory state on IGF-1/GH axis [11].

However, even in the current era of universal NBS, some individuals are diagnosed late, either because they were born before implementation of NBS or in regions in which NBS was not offered, or because of a false-negative NBS. The present study compared the outcome of children with CF who had a LD-CF despite NBS, with children diagnosed after a positive NBS (NBS-CF). The patients with false-negative NBS result and late diagnosis were more stunted and had worse respiratory outcomes including poorer lung function, higher rates of chronic *P. aeruginosa* colonization, and increased frequency of hospitalization for CF-related respiratory illness at follow-up.

In conclusion, as NBS for CF has become universally adopted in the United States and internationally, studies on the early course of disease have become more prevalent. Despite catch-up weight following NBS, linear growth impairment occurs during the first year, even among newborn-screened infants, suggesting that earlier and more aggressive nutritional therapy may be necessary to achieve normal growth. Furthermore, it is clear that lung disease is present in the first months of life, and the ability to change the early course of lung disease in CF has been limited so far. Recent stud-

ies have shown that CFTR modulators that are targeted toward specific CFTR mutations can improve the CFTR function, with resulting improvements in weight and
lung function in adults and older children with CF. These new drug therapies may be
able to prevent the onset of lung disease and other complications of CF if started
early in life; however, safety and efficacy studies in younger children are still to be
completed.

Differences between WHO and CDC early growth measurements in the assessment of cystic fibrosis clinical outcomes

Usatin D[1], Yen EH[1], McDonald C[2], Asfour F[3], Pohl J[4], Robson J[4]

[1]Division of Pediatric Gastroenterology, Hepatology and Nutrition, Department of Pediatrics,
Benioff Children's Hospital, University of California, San Francisco, CA, USA; [2]Primary Children's
Hospital, Salt Lake City, UT, USA; [3]Division of Pediatric Pulmonology, Department of Pediatrics,
Primary Children's Hospital, University of Utah School of Medicine, Salt Lake City, UT, USA; [4] Division
of Pediatric Gastroenterology, Hepatology and Nutrition, Department of Pediatrics, Primary
Children's Hospital, University of Utah School of Medicine, Salt Lake City, UT, USA

J Cyst Fibros 2017;16:503–509

Aims: The study specifically addressed the question whether reaching weight for length (WFL)
≥50th percentile at age 2 years on World Health Organization (WHO) growth standards alone correlates with the same clinical outcomes displayed by those reaching WFL ≥50th percentile on both
WHO and Centers for Disease Control and Prevention (CDC) measures.
Methods: The study included data from the Cystic Fibrosis Foundation Patient Registry (CFFPR)
of children born between 1990 and 1994, diagnosed with CF prior to age 2 years, and followed prospectively. Weight and length taken at the participants' 2-year-old visit were used to calculate WFL.
WFL percentiles were calculated using previously published CDC and WHO algorithms.
Based on the WFL percentiles at the age of 2, the children diagnosed with CF before the age of 2
years were separated into 3 groups: patients <50th percentile on both WHO and CDC measures,
patients achieving ≥50th percentile on the WHO, but not the CDC, and patients achieving ≥50th
percentile on both growth charts.
FEV1 predicted percentage (FEV1pp) and lung transplant-free survival data were tracked annually from early childhood into adulthood. Additional data collected at 18 years were BMI and number of days hospitalized with pulmonary exacerbations in the previous year.
Results: According to the CFFPR 3014/5333, CF patients born between 1990 and 1994 were diagnosed with CF before age 2 years.
CF patients who achieved WFL ≥50th percentile on both WHO and CDC measures at age 2 years
also had the highest FEV1pp at 18 years, compared to those who achieved WFL ≥50th percentile
on the WHO measure alone ($p = 0.041$).
Patients in the categories of WFL <50th percentile on both WHO and CDC or WFL ≥50th percentile on the WHO alone had similar FEV1pp at age 18, both significantly worse than those WFL
≥50th percentile on both the WHO and CDC curves at age 2 years.
Breaking WHO and CDC WFL percentiles at age 2 years into 4 categories: WFL <10th, 10–25th,
25–50th, and ≥50th percentile, showed a stepwise increase in FEV1pp across increasing WFL percentile groupings, for both the WHO and CDC measures.
Lung transplant-free survival at age 18 years was highest among patients who achieved the ≥50th
percentile WFL on both WHO and CDC curves by age 2 years. Similarly, in the adjusted Cox model, lung transplant/mortality risk was lowest in patients who reached WFL ≥50th percentile on both

WHO and CDC measures at age 2 years. Patients with WFL <50th percentile at age 2 years on the WHO and CDC curves had significantly lower BMI at age 18 years than those who achieved ≥50th percentile WFL on both WHO and CDC curves ($p < 0.001$).

Conclusions: This study showed that early growth status is a major predictor of clinical outcomes, including lung function and overall survival, into adulthood. Setting a goal of attaining WFL ≥50th percentile by age 2 years on the CDC curve, not only on WHO curve using intensive treatment with nutritional supplementation, medical therapies and behavioral interventions improve the possibility of reaching these goals.

Comments   In 2015, Machogu et al. [11] published data on pulmonary function outcome at 6 years in 1,155 children with CF from the CFFPR according to their weight for age (WFA) or WFL percentiles at the age of 2 years, evaluated either using WHO or CDC growth charts. The results were straightforward: children with WFL on 50th percentile on WHO charts, who were bellow 50th percentile according to CDC chart, had a lower FEV1 at the age of 6 years compared to children at or above the 50th percentile on both charts. The authors of this study looked further on and reported the pulmonary function and overall survival at age 18 years related to growth data evaluated using WHO or CDC growth charts at 2 years age. Lung function and transplant-free survival at age 18 years was highest among patients who achieved the ≥50th percentile WFL on both WHO and CDC curves by age 2 years.

Use of the WHO standards to measure children from 12 months to 2 years routinely yields higher WFL percentiles compared to the CDC curves in children with CF. WFL measurements using WHO standards at age 2 may generate a false sense of security among providers and families with respect to achievement of early growth goals. This discrepancy has important implications for children diagnosed with CF, as several studies have shown a strong association between early growth and CF clinical outcomes throughout childhood and as shown in this study with long-term survival. Until the ideal/best WHO BMI percentile will be established/validated with long-term outcomes, health providers for CF children should still set up their nutritional goals above ≥50th percentile for WFL/ BMI on CDC growth charts.

Macronutrient intake in preschoolers with cystic fibrosis and the relationship between macronutrients and growth

Filigno SS[1, 2], Robson SM[1, 3], Szczesniak RD[4, 5], Chamberlin LA[1], Baker MA[6], Sullivan SM[1], Kroner J[1], Powers SW[1, 2]

[1]Division of Behavioral Medicine and Clinical Psychology, Cincinnati Children's Hospital Medical Center, Cincinnati, OH, USA; [2]Department of Pediatrics, University of Cincinnati College of Medicine, Cincinnati, OH, USA; [3]Department of Behavioral Health and Nutrition, University of Delaware, DE, USA; [4]Division of Biostatistics and Epidemiology, Cincinnati Children's Hospital Medical Center, Cincinnati, OH, USA; [5]Division of Pulmonary Medicine, Cincinnati Children's Hospital Medical Center, Cincinnati, OH; USA; [6]Vascular Biology Program, Department of Surgery, Boston Children's Hospital, Boston, MA, USA

J Cyst Fibros 2017;16:519–524

Aims: The study investigated the baseline dietary intake of preschoolers, including percentage of children with CF reaching recommended caloric intake and the distribution of macronutrient intake overall and by meal. The relationship of macronutrient intake to growth was also evaluated.

Methods: The study analyzed dietary data from a large multisite randomized clinical trial of preschool-aged children with CF that examined the effectiveness of a behavioral and nutrition intervention compared to an education and control treatment (CONTROL) to improve intake and growth. Participant demographics were collected via a parent completed questionnaire. All anthropometric and dietary measures were taken at baseline and post-treatment (6 months). Dietary intake of each child was assessed using a 7-day dietary record completed by parents. Given there were no significant differences between behavioral and nutrition intervention and CONTROL groups on dietary intake prior to treatment, intake for both treatment groups was collapsed to examine descriptive statistics regarding the overall dietary intake for the entire sample.

Results: The study included 75 children aged 2–6 years diagnosed with CF and PI. The mean (±SD) age was 3.8 (±1.3) and baseline weight for age z-score was –0.41 (±0.80) and height for age (HAZ) was –0.51 (±0.81). BMI was less than the 50th percentile in 44% of children. Compared to the average recommended daily allowances (RDA), the energy intake achieved at baseline was 109.5% (±25.8), with only 45% of all children meeting the 110% minimum RDA recommendation. Only 53% of children were meeting the minimum recommendation of 35% daily energy from fat. Of the 44% of children defined at nutritional risk (<50th BMI percentile), 55% were not meeting the 110% minimum RDA. Children meeting the optimal nutritional status (≥50th BMI percentile) were consuming an average of 94 kcal/kg/day, within the ≥90–110 kcal/kg/day recommendation to sustain growth. Regarding the relationship between macronutrients and growth, change in percent energy from protein was a significant predictor of change in HAZ from baseline to post-treatment, $F(1125) = 12.93$, $p < 0.001$. Change in percent energy from fat or carbohydrates did not significantly impact change in HAZ or weight for age z-score.

Conclusions: The results of this study showed that many preschool children were not meeting nutrition and growth recommendations for children with CF. Increasing intake of macronutrients with a great impact on energy intake and growth should be a primary nutritional target. Interventions to increase nutrition intake should include tracking and monitoring of macronutrients in addition to total energy and thorough growth monitoring.

Comments According to CFF nutrition consensus and guidelines, children and adolescents with CF are expected to experience typical growth when appropriate nutrition and PERT are provided [13, 14]. Close attention to nutrition and growth is integral to the care of patients with CF and should be assessed at every visit. Nutritional status by all parameters (wasting, stunting, body composition) has been shown to affect lung function and survival in patients with CF in many studies before and this year too [15]. Despite close monitoring and appropriate anticipatory guidance, BMI greater than the 50th percentile can be difficult to attain and maintain. The nutritional status in children with CF has been improving over time, however, on average BMI percentile decreases with advancing age.

Nutritional care of patients with CF should address several aspects including: provision of appropriate amount of calories, PERT, and fat-soluble vitamin supplementation. Achieving the recommended caloric intake of 110–200% of the RDA of kcal/kg with at least 35–40% of daily energy derived from fat in children with CF is sometimes difficult. This study reported the nutritional data of a contemporary sample of preschoolers receiving standard of care at several accredited CF Centers in the US.

The reported data is not encouraging as more than half (55%) of the preschoolers were not meeting the minimum 110% RDA for energy recommendation, and 44% of children had BMIs <50th percentile. The average daily percent energy from fat consumed for the entire sample was just at the minimum recommendation of 35%, and

Hartman · Shamir

only 53% of the children were meeting this recommendation. Children were within the acceptable macronutrient distribution range for carbohydrates and protein.

The increased focus on improving the nutritional status in patients with CF over the last years has contributed to more children receiving proactive assessment and intervention. An approach to feeding education during the preschool years involves systematic monitoring, goal setting, and timely feedback about nutrition intake that can help parents of children with CF to engage in feeding practices with the goal of achieving optimal nutrition outcomes. A variety of options are available for the management of suboptimal nutritional status, including oral supplementation (vitamin and mineral supplementation and calorie-dense liquids), behavioral treatment, pharmacotherapy (including appetite stimulants and CFTR modulators), and enteral nutrition. Awareness of clinical staff about the overall nutritional status of their patient population and timely nutritional support when clinical indices fall below standards should be the standard of care.

Celiac Disease

Celiac disease is associated with reduced bone mineral density and increased FRAX scores in the US National Health and Nutrition Examination survey

Kamycheva E[1–3], Goto T[1, 4], Camargo CA Jr[1, 4]

[1]Department of Emergency Medicine, Massachusetts General Hospital, Harvard Medical School, Boston, MA 02114, USA; [2]Medical Clinic, University Hospital of North Norway, Tromsoe, Norway; [3]Endocrine Research Group, Faculty of Health Sciences, Department of Clinical Medicine, UiT The Arctic University of Norway, Tromsoe, Norway; [4]Harvard T.H. Chan School of Public Health, Boston, MA, USA

Osteoporosis Int 2017;28:781–790

Aims: National Health and Nutrition Examination Survey (NHANES) is a unique program of studies designed to assess the health and nutritional status of US adults and children. The survey combines interviews and physical examinations of about 5,000 persons per year. Based on the most recent nationally representative NHANES datasets from cycles 2009–2010 to 2013–2014, the study investigated whether CD is associated with decreased bone mineral density (BMD) and is an independent risk factor of osteoporotic fractures in the US population.

Methods: The NHANES data included questionnaire data (diet and behavior), tissue transglutaminase IgA (tTG IgA) and anthropometry. CD was defined by positive (>10.0 U/mL) or weakly positive (4.0–10.0 U/mL) tTG IgA ELISA test. BMD of hip and spine was measured by dual energy X-ray absorptiometry (DXA). DXA scans were performed on eligible survey participants 8 years and older during the 2009–2010 cycle and only on participants aged ≥40 years during 2013–2014 NHANES cycle. Fracture risk assessment tool (FRAX) score (10-year risk for hip fracture and major osteoporotic fractures, hip, clinical spine, wrist, and humerus) was calculated for participants aged ≥40 years.

Results: NHANES, 2009–2010 included 6,712 individuals, 1,466 children 6–18 years old. Using the linear regression model with multiple adjustments (for serum 25-hydroxyvitamin D [25(OH)D], vitamin D-containing supplements, calcium-containing supplements, and smoking status), BMD z-scores for hip were found to be significantly lower for children with CD (Δ z-score -0.59, $p = 0.02$). BMD z-scores for spine were also significantly lower in children with CD (Δ z-score -0.46, $p < 0.001$) as compared to children without CD. In adults aged $\geq$18 years, only men with CD tended to have lower BMD in hip by 0.06 g/cm^2 ($p = 0.08$); they also demonstrated lower BMD in spine by 0.11 g/cm^2 ($p < 0.001$), as compared to men without CD.

NHANES, 2013–2014 included 2,993 adults 40 years and older. In the linear regression model (adjusted for BMI, serum calcium, intake of milk, and smoking status), men with CD had 0.14 g/cm^2 lower BMD for hip ($p = 0.02$) and 0.11 g/cm^2 lower BMD for spine ($p = 0.005$), as compared to their counterparts without CD. Moreover, men with CD had 2.25 % higher FRAX hip fracture score ($p = 0.006$) and 2.43% higher FRAX major fracture score ($p = 0.05$), as compared to men without CD. By contrast, there was no difference in BMD or FRAX scores among women with and without CD.

Conclusions: This nationally representative database of the US population reports a significant association between CD/ CD autoimmunity and reduced BMD in both children and male adults. Furthermore, in men aged $\geq$40 years, CD/CD autoimmunity was significantly associated with higher FRAX fracture score and, thus, appears to be an independent risk factor for osteoporotic fractures in this group.

However, the study' findings only pertain to subjects with CD autoimmunity. The presence of CD was not validated by either duodenal biopsies or patient's medical records. Thus, subjects with known CD adherent to gluten-free diet (GFD) were not included in the CD group. Nevertheless, assuming that subjects included in the CD group could have undiagnosed CD, or are diagnosed but not adhering to GFD, the results are of major clinical importance: (1) to promote active screening and diagnosis for CD and (2) adherence to GFD in patients already diagnosed with CD.

Reduced bone mineral density in children with screening-detected celiac disease

Björck S[1], Brundin C[1], Karlsson M[2], Agardh D[1]

[1]Unit of Diabetes and Celiac Disease, Department of Clinical Sciences, Malmö, Lund University, Sweden, [2]Clinical and Molecular Osteoporosis Research Unit, Department of Clinical Sciences and Orthopedics, Lund University, Sweden

J Pediatr Gastroenterol Nutr 2017;65:526–532

Aims: The aim of this study was to evaluate if BMD is affected in children with asymptomatic, screening detected CD either with or without GFD.

Methods: The study evaluated children participating in the Celiac Disease Prediction in Skåne (CiPiS) study, a prospective population-based cohort study aimed to identify CD by repeated screening using tTG IgA in HLA genotyped children. At the age of 9 years, children participating in the CiPiS were invited for measurement of BMD and bone-related metabolites.

The study investigated 3 cohorts selected from the CiPiS study:

1 Children diagnosed with CD at 3 years age, 56/3,435, based on positive tTG IgA blood test and intestinal biopsy who were on GFD at the time of investigation

2 Children diagnosed with CD at 9 years age, 72/4,077, by and additional tTG IgA screening, before initiation of GFD

3 A control group matched for gender, HLA-DQ, and birth year for every child with CD was selected from the tTG IgA negative children at follow-up screening.

All participants were investigated by anthropometry, a questionnaire related to lifestyle factors, BMD, and a blood sample for evaluation of different parameters related to bone mineral metabolism.

Results: Lifestyle parameters were not different between the 3 study groups with the exception of GFD in the cohort diagnosed with CD at the age of 3 years.

BMD: Compared to controls, the 9 year old children with screening-detected CD had lower total body and spine BMD at diagnosis. Children diagnosed with CD at 3 years, and on GFD had no different BMD when compared to controls.

25(OH) Vitamin D3 and PTH: 25(OH)D3 levels were lower and PTH levels were higher in untreated newly diagnosed CD children, compared to controls. Children with CD on GFD did not differ from control in levels of 25(OH)D3 and PTH.

Systemic cytokines: In children newly diagnosed with CD, systemic levels of the cytokines IL-1β, IL-6, IL-8, IL-10, IL12p70, IL-13, and TNFα were increased in spite of levels of IL-15 were decreased compared to matched controls. Children on GFD did not differ from controls in any measured systemic cytokine.

Conclusions: Asymptomatic children 9 years old with screening-detected CD had lower total body and spine BMD already at diagnosis, whereas children with CD on GFD had BMD similar to healthy controls. This strengthens the conclusion that children with CD diagnosed by population-based screening, may benefit from an early diagnosis to institute treatment to restore bone health.

At-risk screened children with Celiac disease are comparable in disease severity and dietary adherence to those found because of clinical suspicion: a large cohort study

Kivelä L[1], Kaukinen K[2, 3], Huhtala H[4], Lähdeaho ML[1], Mäki M[1], Kurppa K[1]

[1]Tampere Center for Child Health Research, University of Tampere and Tampere University Hospital, Tampere, Finland; [2]School of Medicine, University of Tampere, Tampere, Finland; [3]Department of Internal Medicine, Tampere University Hospital, Tampere, Finland; [4]Tampere School of Health Sciences, University of Tampere, Tampere, Finland

J Pediatr 2017;183:115–121.e2

Aims: The study aimed to identify clinical, serologic, and histological features and follow-up results in a high-risk group of children diagnosed with CD by screening and compare it with those identified based on clinical suspicion, and thus evaluate the potential benefits and detriments of CD screening.

Methods: The study analyzed the data collected from the research database at Tampere Center for Child Health Research, University of Tampere and the Department of Pediatrics, Tampere University Hospital, which contains medical information on children diagnosed with CD from the late 1960s to present. The information included patients' clinical characteristics, CD serology, laboratory parameters, severity of histologic damage, and follow-up data regarding adherence and clinical and serologic response to GFD. From 2012 onward, most patients included in the database were participants in a prospective study enrolment. Only children diagnosed from the year 2000 onward were included. Altogether, 504 children with CD proven by biopsy were included in the final study cohort.

Results: Of the children included in the analysis, 145 (28.8%) were detected by screening and 359 (71.2%) based on symptoms (gastrointestinal in 68.0% and extra-intestinal in 32.0%). However, 51.8% of the screening-detected children reported symptoms at diagnosis, usually less severe than in patients diagnosed clinically, but otherwise the groups did not differ in the distribution of symptoms. Anemia (7.1 vs. 22.9%, $p < 0.001$), poor growth (15.7 vs 36.9%, $p < 0.001$) were more prevalent in clinically based diagnosed children. Hb (126 vs. 124 g/L, $p = 0.008$) and albumin (41.0 vs. 38.0

g/L, $p = 0.016$) were lower in clinically detected patients. There were no differences in serology or histology between the groups. Screening-detected children had better dietary adherence (91.2 vs. 83.2%, $p = 0.047$). The groups showed equal clinical response (97.5 vs. 96.2%, $p = 0.766$) to GFD.

Conclusions: More than half of the screening-detected patients with CD had symptoms unrecognized at diagnosis. The severity of histologic damage, antibody levels, dietary adherence, and response to treatment in screening-detected cases was comparable with those detected on a clinical basis. The results of the study show that even apparently asymptomatic patients may have well advanced serologic and histologic disease and therefore a subsequent risk of long-term complications.

Comments   CD is an autoimmune enteropathy that develops in genetically predisposed individuals, upon ingestion of gluten, the major storage protein in wheat, barley, and rye.

The common presentation of CD has shifted from the historically classic symptoms of malabsorption (chronic diarrhea, weight loss, and failure to thrive) in childhood to non-classic symptoms, which can be present in childhood or adulthood. The more common, non-classical symptoms include iron deficiency, bloating, constipation, chronic fatigue, headache, abdominal pain, and osteoporosis.

CD can affect the bone health of children in several ways and present with a variety of signs and symptoms including bone pain, rickets, tetany, osteomalacia, osteopenia, osteoporosis, fractures associated with minimal trauma, or growth failure with or without symptoms of malabsorption. With the exception of osteopenia or osteoporosis identified by DXA, other manifestations are rarely the presenting signs and symptoms of CD in children [17].

Most reports of low BMD are from symptomatic patients diagnosed with CD. Timely diagnosis and initiation of a GFD rapidly restores bone mass to normal levels in children and adolescents [18]. Instruction on age-appropriate intake of calcium, vitamin D, and the need for exercise to promote bone health should be provided during nutritional counseling at the time of diagnosis.

Albeit screening-detected children have similar degree of mucosal damage than those diagnosed based on clinical suspicion, whether screening-detected children have reduced BMD as a consequence of an unrecognized disease already present at diagnosis has not been shown. The study of Sara Björck investigated for the presence of low BMD in asymptomatic children prospectively identified in a population-based screening compared to matched controls diagnosed with CD 6 years before and on GFD and children without CD. The study found that children with screening-detected CD had lower total body and spine BMD already at 9 years of age whereas children with already screening-detected CD on GFD since early age had a BMD similar to healthy controls. The study adds to the arguments that children detected in population-based screening, may benefit from an early diagnosis to institute GFD to restore bone health.

The NHANES-based study of Kamycheva described in this chapter on page 99, investigated the association between CD autoimmunity (positive serology) and BMD (children and men ≥18 years) and increased risk of fractures in men ≥40 years. In this study, CD was defined as positive tTG IgA test, a test with sensitivity of 93% and specificity of more than 98%. The study identified a significant association between CD autoimmunity and reduced BMD in both children and adults. Furthermore, in men aged ≥40 years, CD autoimmunity was significantly associated with FRAX hip fracture score and borderline significantly associated with FRAX major fracture score and, thus, appears to be an independent risk factor for osteoporotic fractures in men. This study, therefore, suggests that not only asymptomatic children with CD, but also children and adults with positive celiac serology/ autoimmunity are at risk of poor bone status and osteoporotic-related fractures in adulthood.

Hartman · Shamir

CD fulfils several WHO criteria for population screening, although the benefits of this approach remain controversial, in particular, because it is unclear whether asymptomatic screening-detected patients will adhere to the demanding and restrictive GFD and whether clinical outcome of these patients is similar to those detected due to malabsorptive symptoms. Although untreated CD predisposes to severe complications in symptomatic patients, it is not known whether this is also true to screening-detected individuals with possible less severe histologic damage. The previous 2 studies showed that low bone mass have been detected even in otherwise asymptomatic children with CD, and even in individuals with positive celiac autoimmunity, and this situation may remain permanent if left untreated.

This study investigated the clinical, serologic, histologic features and follow-up results in children with CD diagnosed during screening in a risk group and those identified based on clinical suspicion. The authors reported a high prevalence of unrecognized gastrointestinal symptoms as well as anemia and poor growth. Furthermore, the severity of histologic damage, antibody levels, dietary adherence, and response to treatment in screening-detected cases was comparable with those detected on a clinical basis.

The results of this study and the previous ones suggest that based on the high percentage of unrecognized clinical symptoms and excellent response, adherence to the GFD active screening for CD is highly recommended. Alternatively, a low-threshold case finding among at-risk children should be adopted, but it is important to realize that even apparently asymptomatic patients may have well advanced serologic and histologic disease and a subsequent risk of long-term complications.

Early growth in children with celiac disease: a cohort study

Kahrs CR[1,2], Magnus MC[3–5], Stigum H[3], Lundin KEA[6,7], Størdal K[1,2]

[1]Department of Pediatrics, Østfold Hospital Trust, Grålum, Norway, [2]Department of Child Health, Norwegian Institute of Public Health, Oslo, Norway; [3]Department of NonCommunicable Diseases, Norwegian Institute of Public Health, Oslo, Norway; [4]MRC Integrative Epidemiology Unit, University of Bristol, Bristol, UK; [5]School of Social and Community Medicine, University of Bristol, Bristol, UK; [6]Department of Gastroenterology, Oslo University Hospital Rikshospitalet, Oslo, Norway; [7]Centre for Immune Regulation, University of Oslo, Oslo, Norway

Arch Dis Child 2017;102:1037–1043

Aims: The study investigated growth during the first 2 years of life in children later diagnosed with CD compared with children without CD.

Methods: The Norwegian Mother and Child Cohort Study is a prospective population-based pregnancy cohort study conducted by the Norwegian Institute of Public Health. The children evaluated in the present study were born from 1999 to 2009. The children's weight and length at birth and at 3, 6, 8, 12, 15–18, and 24 months were used for the present study. CD was identified through combined data from the questionnaires administered to parents and the Norwegian Patient Register.

Results: The study enrolled 58,235 cohort controls and 440 children with CD. The mean age at the end of follow-up was 8.6 years (range 4.6–14.2).

Height: The longitudinal analysis for the period 0–12 months yielded a non-significant reduction in height z-score for children with CD, whereas the period 0–24 months yielded a significant reduction (–0.07 SD scores (SDS) per year, 95% CI –0.13 to –0.01), as compared with children without CD.

Weight: The longitudinal analysis from 0 to 12 months yielded no significant differences for weight among children with CD versus controls at the end of follow-up, with similar non-significant differences from 0 to 24 months of age (–0.01 SDS, 95% CI –0.08 to –0.05).

Conclusions: Children later diagnosed with CD were shorter as early as 12 months of age compared with those without diagnosis at the end of follow-up. The differences in absolute numbers were small at 12 months but increased in the second year of life even when excluding children with symptoms from before 2 years of age. As symptoms started at a mean of 4 years, the study suggests that growth impairment occur early and commonly in children with CD.

Comments   Recent studies have reported a decrease in the prevalence of failure to thrive and short stature as presenting manifestation of CD, to 26 and 11% respectively. Growth failure has been reported to be present 1 (boys) and even 2 (girls) years prior to the diagnosis of CD. Several studies have shown that the institution of GFD in children with newly diagnosed CD leads to rapid symptoms' disappearance and catch-up of body weight (mostly within the first year after withdrawal of the gluten from the diet) whereas height catches up somewhat more gradually, sometimes up to 2–3 years or even more.

The study of Kahrs CR reported that growth faltering occurred even in the first 2 years of life, long before the symptoms or diagnosis of CD was done. There was no knowledge of CD serology at that time in these children, but it is possible that GH-IGF-1 axis disturbance was present at that time, even before CD serology seroconversion, at the earliest stages of mucosal changes. Prospective studies in children at genetic risk, including thorough investigation of the GH-IGF1 axis will be able to provide new data on the earliest CD-induced systemic changes of growth axis.

Food Allergy

The impact of the elimination diet on growth and nutrient intake in children with food protein induced gastrointestinal allergies

Meyer R[1], De Koker C[2], Dziubak R[1], Godwin H[1], Dominguez-Ortega G[3], Chebar Lozinsky A[4], Skrapac AK[2], Gholmie Y[5], Reeve K[1], Shah N[1, 6]

[1]Gastroenterology Department, Great Ormond Street Hospital for Children NHS foundation Trust, London, UK; [2]Department of Nutrition and Dietetics, Chelsea and Westminster Hospital NHS Foundation Trust, London, UK; [3]Niño Jesús University Children Hospital, Madrid, Spain; [4]Paediatric Gastroenterology, Universidade Federal de Sao Paulo (UNIFESP), São Paulo, Brazil; [5]Department of Nutrition and Food Sciences, Faculty of Agricultural and Food Sciences, American University of Beirut, Beirut, Lebanon; [6]Institute of Child Health, University College, London, UK

Clin Transl Allergy 2016;6:25

Background: Non-IgE mediated food allergies include food protein induced gastrointestinal allergies such as proctocolitis, enterocolitis, eosinophilic gastrointestinal disorders, food protein induced enterocolitis syndrome, and enteropathy. Previous studies have indicated growth faltering in children with IgE-mediated allergy, but limited data is available on those with delayed type allergies. The study reported the impact on growth before and after the start of elimination diets in children with food protein induced non-IgE mediated gastrointestinal allergies.

Methods: This prospective, observational study was performed at the Gastroenterology Department, Great Ormond Street Hospital for Children NHS Foundation Trust, London, UK and enrolled children aged 4 weeks to 16 years without non-allergic comorbidities who were required to follow an elimination diet for the diagnosis of suspected non-IgE mediated gastrointestinal food allergies. Growth data were recorded as z-scores for weight-for-age (Wtage), Htage, and weight-for-height (WtHt) for children ≤5 years of age and BMI for children >5 years. Dietary intake was recorded for a minimum of 4 weeks after initiating the elimination diet.

Results: The study reported the data from 130 children, median age 23.3 months (IQR 9.4–69.2). Hydrolyzed formula (HF) was given to 10.8% children, 17.2% avoided one food, 30.2% 2 foods, 15.5% 3 foods, and 37.1% eliminated ≥4 foods. Almost all children (94.8%) in this study eliminated CM from their diet, 74% also avoided soya with 45.7 and 44.8% avoiding eggs and wheat, respectively. The most frequent combination (30.2%) of eliminated foods was CM, soya, eggs and wheat (with or without other foods).

Anthropometry: The mean Wtage, Htage, WtHt (<5 years of age), and BMI z-scores (>5 years of age) for children after a minimum of 4 weeks elimination was 0.044, –0.186, 0.296, and 0.042. Eleven out of 130 children (9%) were stunted and 2/90 (2.2%) children <5 years of age were wasted (z-score less than –2), and 2/40 (5%) >5 years had a BMI less than –2 z-score. Conversely, 2/90 (2.2%) and 4/40 (10%) children <5 and >5 years of age, respectively, were overweight with a WtHt or BMI z-score >2.

Food intake: Diaries from 110 children were included in the data analysis as some infants were being breastfed. Compared to UK Dietary Reference Values, 68.2 and 50.0% of children met their requirements for energy and protein, respectively. About 21.8% did not achieve their EAR for energy versus only 2.7% not achieving requirements for protein, in fact, 47.3% exceeded the protein requirements for their age.

Association between growth parameters and nutritional intake: There was a statistically significant improvement in Wtage after the 4-week elimination diet. The elimination diet itself (i.e., CM, soya, egg, wheat) and the number of foods eliminated did not have a positive impact on growth over a 4-week period. However, vitamin and/or mineral supplements and hypoallergenic formulas were positively associated with WtHt and Wtage.

Conclusions: Nutritional management of children with non-IgE mediated gastrointestinal food allergies, significantly impacts growth. In this study, patients had improved growth parameters (weight) following dietary elimination. This positive impact was associated with energy and protein intake, the use of HF and vitamin and/or mineral supplementation, irrespective of the type of elimination diet and the numbers of foods eliminated. Whether these findings are unique to children with this type of allergy and stable over a longer period of diet elimination should be studied further.

Iodine status and growth in 0- to 2-year-old infants with cow's milk protein allergy

Thomassen RA[1], Kvammen JA[1], Eskerud MB[2], Júlíusson PB[3], Henriksen C[4], Rugtveit J[1]

[1]Department of Paediatric Medicine, Division of Paediatric and Adolescent Medicine, Oslo University Hospital, Oslo, Norway; [2]Department of Internal Medicine, Clinical Nutrition, Lovisenberg Diaconal Hospital, Oslo, Norway; [3]Department of Clinical Science, University of Bergen, Bergen, Norway; [4]Department of Nutrition, Institute of Basic Medical Sciences, Faculty of Medicine, University of Oslo, Norway

J Pediatr Gastroenterol Nutr 2017;64:806–811

Background: Iodine is an essential trace element necessary for the production of thyroid hormones, and adequate levels of thyroid hormones are needed for normal growth and neurological development of the brain and central nervous system in infancy and childhood. Several case reports have found goiter and signs of goiter due to low iodine intake in children restricting cow's milk protein (CMP) in their diet. The aim of the present study was to investigate iodine intake and status and growth in CMP allergic (CMPA) children and identify factors affecting iodine status and growth.

Methods: This observational cross-sectional study included 57 infants less than 2 years of age with CMPA. Two spot urine samples were collected and analyzed for iodine, together with a 3-day food record and a food frequency questionnaire. Urine iodine concentrations were compared with the WHO cut-off values for iodine deficiency (median urinary iodine concentration [MUIC] of >100 mg/L is considered as adequate in children younger than 2 years). SDS of weight, length, and head circumference at birth and at study inclusion were recorded.

Results: The median age was 9 months and the median time on CMP-free diet before enrolment was 17 weeks. Almost all children (98%) had gastrointestinal symptoms, 46% had eczema or skin symptoms, more than one third had failure to thrive and one third had food refusal. Feeding difficulties were reported in 70% of the children. More than half (57%) were breastfed at the time of enrolment; 24% mainly breastfed and 33% partially. An HA was used by 69%. MUIC was 159 µg/L (<25–457 µg/L) and the prevalence of MUIC <100 µg/L was 31%. The mainly breastfed children had significantly higher prevalence of iodine deficiency: 58% had a MUIC <100 µg/L compared with 12 and 32% in the partially breastfed and the weaned. The total iodine intake and percentage of RDI for iodine (excluding breast milk) was significantly higher in the partially breastfed and weaned children compared to the mainly breastfed children. The dietary factors positively associated with iodine excretion were enriched baby cereals and meeting the dietary requirement for iodine. Stunting was present in 5%. Underweight and wasting in 11% and were associated with food refusal and poor appetite, but not with iodine status.

Conclusions: The present study suggests that children with CMPA have a high prevalence of iodine deficiency and slightly lower growth deficit than the reference population; however, the 2 conditions were not related. The mainly breastfed infants were at higher risk of iodine deficiency compared to weaned infants on HF or consuming enriched baby cereals. The children with feeding difficulties had increased risk of malnutrition.

Comments Food allergies are commonly diagnosed in children, and recent statistics show an increasing worldwide prevalence of reported food allergies. Food allergies affect approximately 8% of children and 5% of adults [19]. Allergen avoidance is the mainstay of treatment for food allergy; however, many of the most common food allergens are integral parts of the typical Western diet and contain macronutrients and micronutrients that are essential for normal growth and development. Even with close supervision, growth in children with food allergy can lag. Although several studies have assessed the relationship of food allergy, nutrition, and growth in smaller groups of children, population-wide studies investigating these issues are limited [20]. Cow's milk allergy (CMA) represents the most common food allergy during childhood, affecting 2–3% of children. A strict elimination diet removing cow's milk, dairy products, and their traces remains the main treatment plan until allergy resolution.

One of the largest studies that examined growth status in children with food allergies included 6,189 children aged 2–17 years from NHANES 2007–2008 and 2009–2010. Overall, 6.3% (95% CI 5.5–7.3) of children reported a food allergy, with the most common trigger identified as milk (1.8%; 95% CI 1.3–2.3), followed by peanut (1.2%; 95% CI 0.9–1.6) and egg (0.6%; 95% CI 0.4–0.8). In multivariate analyses, mean weight, height, and BMI percentiles were significantly lower in those with milk allergy but not in other groups of children with food allergy. Children with milk allergy also had decreased triceps skin folds, a measurement of adiposity (mean difference, 1.8 mm; 95% CI 0.55–3.05 mm; $p = 5.006$). Adjustment for dietary intake of total calories, protein, fat, calcium, and vitamin D did not change the findings of decreased growth measurements in children with milk allergy or adiposity measurements [21]. What the NHANES study reinforces is that in a non-IgE mediated gastrointestinal allergy population on an elimination diet, a significant number of children with this allergy will be stunted, irrespective of dietary advice including a suitable hydrolyzed formula and vitamin and mineral supplementation.

The study of Meyer et al., described above in page 104, investigated the change in weight and height after a minimum of 4 weeks elimination diet (for 94.8% cow's milk elimination) in 110 children aged 23.3 months (IQR 9.4–69.2) with non-IgE mediated milk allergy. The study showed improvement in WtHt and Wtage on the elimination diet, unrelated to the elimination diet itself (i.e. CM, soya, egg, wheat) and the number of foods eliminated. In this study, stunting was present in 9% of children, but only a very small number of children were wasted (2.2 and 5%). As there was on average a minimum of 4 weeks between the start of the elimination diet and the follow-up measurements, the time was insufficient for significant linear growth to occur. The study shows that individualized dietary advice may help children with non-IgE mediated gastrointestinal food allergies on elimination diet maintain and even improve the weight. Whether height could also be improved in these children should be investigated over longer period times.

The study of iodine status in infants with CMPA and children on CMP free diets reported a poor iodine status in infants on exclusive breast milk compared to infants on combined breast milk and formula or formula only. However, the iodine status in the CMPA infants in the current study was a cross-sectional one without a control group and was not inferior compared with healthy infants in other iodine sufficient countries and the data on iodine status of healthy infants in Norway are lacking. Moreover, despite the slightly lower mean weight SDS and length SDS for the study population, there was no correlation between growth and iodine deficiency in this cohort.

Since breastfed infants are highly dependent on the content of iodine in breast milk, which in turn is dependent on the breastfeeding mothers' iodine status, breastfeeding mothers should be monitored and dietary advice on iodine sources and supplements should be offered. The relationship between growth and iodine status in infants on exclusive breastfeeding should be further investigated.

The effect of food allergies and food avoidance on children's health should include not only comprehensive dietary advice and follow-up to ensure appropriate macro- and micronutrients' intake and normal growth pattern but also timely achievement of appropriate feeding skills and behavior.

Association of stimulant medication use with bone mass in children and adolescents with attention-deficit/hyperactivity disorder

Feuer AJ[1], Thai A[2], Demmer RT[2], Vogiatzi M[3]

[1]Division of Pediatric Endocrinology and Diabetes, Weill Cornell Medicine, New York, NY, USA;
[2]Department of Epidemiology, Mailman School of Public Health, Columbia University Medical Center, New York, NY, USA [3]Division of Pediatric Endocrinology and Diabetes, The Children's Hospital of Philadelphia, Philadelphia, Pennsylvania, PA, USA

JAMA Pediatr 2016;170:e162804

Background and aims: Animal studies suggest that sympathetic nervous system activation leads to decreased bone mass. Stimulant medications used to treat attention-deficit/hyperactivity disorder (ADHD) have been shown to decrease growth velocity in pediatric patients, but their effect on bone mass is not clear. Since amphetamines increase sympathetic tone, it is possible that they also affect bone remodeling. Because bone mass accrual takes place during childhood and adolescence, assessment of stimulant medications' effects on bone density in growing children is of critical importance. The present study investigated the association between stimulant use and bone mass in children and adolescents.

Methods: This cross-sectional analysis used data collected from January 1, 2005, to December 31, 2010, from the NHANES database. NHANES is a series of cross-sectional, nationally representative health and nutrition surveys of the US population. All children, adolescents, and young adults aged 8–20 years with DXA, anthropometric, demographic, and prescription medication data were eligible for participation. Stimulant users were defined as participants who reported use of amphetamine, methylphenidate, lisdexamfetamine dimesylate, dextroamphetamine sulfate, or levoamphetamine. Nonusers were defined as participants who did not report the use of those medications. Of the 6,489 respondents included in the multivariable linear regression analysis, 159 were stimulant users and 6,330 were nonusers. Bone mineral content (BMC) and BMD were measured using DXA scans of the left hip and lumbar spine. Demographic variables included age, sex, and race or ethnicity, anthropometry (height, weight, BMI z-scores, smoking status, physical activity, and socioeconomic status as well as serum levels of 25(OH)D were related to BMD and BMC measurements.

Results: The study included 6,489 NHANES participants with a mean (±SD) age of 13.6 (±3.6) years. There were 159 individuals who reported stimulant use.

Male users had significantly lower BMIs, BMI z scores, weight, and weight z scores than nonusers, whereas female stimulant users had significantly lower weight and BMI. Male and female users had significantly shorter heights than nonusers. The poverty income ratio and physical activity level were similar in both groups. Serum 25(OH)D concentrations were significantly higher among stimulant users versus nonusers.

Stimulant use was still associated with lower bone mass after adjustment for covariates. The mean lumbar spine BMC was significantly lower in stimulant users versus nonusers (12.76 g; 95% CI 12.28–13.27 vs. 13.38 g; 95% CI 13.26–13.51 g; $p = 0.02$), as was the mean lumbar spine BMD (0.90 g/cm^2; 95% CI 0.87–0.94 vs. 0.94 g/cm^2; 95% CI 0.94–0.94 g/cm^2; $p - 0.03$) and mean femoral neck BMC (4.34 g; 95% CI 4.13–4.57 vs. 4.59 g; 95% CI 4.56–4.62 g; $p = 0.03$). The mean BMD of the femoral neck (0.88 g/cm^2; 95% CI 0.84–0.91 vs. 0.91 g/cm^2; 95% CI 0.90–0.91 g/cm^2; $p = 0.08$) and total femur (0.94 g/cm^2; 95% CI 0.90–0.99 vs. 0.99 g/cm^2; 95% CI 0.98–0.99 g/cm^2; $p = 0.05$) were also lower in stimulant users versus nonusers. Participants treated with stimulants for 3 months or longer had significantly lower lumbar spine BMD (0.89 g/cm^2; 95% CI 0.85–0.93 vs. 0.94 g/cm^2; 95% CI 0.94–0.94 g/cm^2; $p = 0.02$) and BMC (12.71 g; 95% CI 12.14–13.32 vs. 13.38 g; 95% CI 13.25–13.51 g; $p = 0.03$) and femoral neck BMD (0.87 g/cm^2; 95% CI 0.74–0.83 vs. 0.91 g/cm^2; 95% CI 0.83–0.84 g/cm^2; $p = 0.048$) than nonusers.

Conclusions: The use of stimulants in children and adolescents was associated with lower DXA measurements of the lumbar spine and femur compared with nonusers. Reduction in bone mass during the critical period of bone accrual in adolescence and early adulthood can lead to permanent reduction in bone density and increase the risk of fractures. The study findings support the need for future prospective studies to examine the effects of stimulant use on bone mass in children.

Comments ADHD is one of the commonly diagnosed childhood neurodevelopmental disorders, affecting around 3–4% of children and adolescents [23]. ADHD is characterized by age-inappropriate symptoms of inattention, hyperactivity, and impulsivity. Stimulant medications such as methylphenidate and dexamphetamine are the first-line pharmacological treatment of ADHD. The short-term evidence base efficacy of stimulants is well established. However, its long-term benefits are still unclear. While serious adverse events are very rare, common adverse effects include sleep disturbances, loss of appetite, and reduced growth.

Amphetamines are classified as indirect sympathomimetic agents that activate peripheral β-adrenergic receptors. During normal bone remodeling, norepinephrine suppresses bone formation and stimulates bone resorption, an effect that is mediated by the β2-adrenergic receptors expressed by osteoblasts. Because amphetamines increase β-adrenergic signaling, they may exert detrimental effects on the growing skeleton. Mice with β-adrenergic receptor knockout display a high bone mass phenotype. Furthermore, mice and adults with β-adrenergic blocking have higher BMD, suggesting that β-adrenergic signaling may also affect bone remodeling and bone mass in humans [24].

The effects of stimulants on bone have not been well studied. Using the NHANES extensive data, the present study shows that use of stimulants in children and adolescents was associated with significantly lower mean lumbar spine BMD and BMC and lower femoral neck BMC and total femur BMD. Noteworthy, BMD and BMC results were adjusted according to height and BMI z-scores which are important variables in the interpretation of DXA results in children. Since childhood and adolescence are critical periods of bone accrual, the lower bone mass in stimulant users is likely to be of clinical importance as longitudinal tracking of DXA measurements indicates that skeletal status during childhood is a strong predictor of peak bone mass in young adulthood [25]. Furthermore, a 5% to 10% reduction in peak BMD (equivalent to a reduction of BMD from 0.5 to 1 SD) can substantially increase the incidence of future fractures. As the prevalence of ADHD increases and the rate of ADHD diagnoses rise, the prescriptions for stimulants dispensed for these children are also in rise. As with other long-term concerns regarding the use of stimulants, including their possible effects on cardiovascular health and the risk of inducing other psychiatric problems, the skeletal effect and future risk for fracture should be further investigated [26].

References

1 Gasparetto M, Guariso G: Crohn's disease and growth deficiency in children and adolescents. World J Gastroenterol 2014;20:13219–13233.

2 Hyams J, Crandall W, Kugathasan S, et al; REACH Study Group: Induction and maintenance infliximab therapy for the treatment of moderate-to-severe Crohn's disease in children. Gastroenterology 2007; 132:863–873.

3 Goodhand JR, Kamperidis N, Rao A, et al: Prevalence and management of anemia in children, adolescents, and adults with inflammatory bowel disease. Inflamm Bowel Dis 2012;18:513–519.

4 Nemeth E, Tuttle MS, Powelson J, et al: Hepcidin regulates cellular iron efflux by binding to ferroportin and inducing its internalization. Science 2004; 306:2090–2093.

5 Fraenkel PG: Anemia of inflammation: a review. Med Clin North Am 2017;101:285–296.

6 Murawska N, Fabisiak A, Fichna J: Anemia of chronic disease and iron deficiency anemia in inflammatory bowel diseases: pathophysiology, diagnosis, and treatment. Inflamm Bowel Dis 2016;22:1198–1208.

7 Dignass AU, Gasche C, Bettenworth D, et al; European Crohn's and Colitis Organisation [ECCO]: European consensus on the diagnosis and management of iron deficiency and anaemia in inflammatory bowel diseases. J Crohns Colitis 2015;9:211–222.

8 Danielson BG: Structure, chemistry, and pharmacokinetics of intravenous iron agents. J Am Soc Nephrol 2004;15(suppl 2):S93–S98.

9 Kulnigg S, Stoinov S, Simanenkov V, et al: A novel intravenous iron formulation for treatment of anemia in inflammatory bowel disease: the ferric carboxymaltose (FERINJECT) randomized controlled trial. Am J Gastroenterol 2008;103:1182–1192.

10 Castellani C, Massie J, Sontag M, Southern KW: Newborn screening for cystic fibrosis. Lancet Respir Med 2016;4:653–661.

11 Laursen EM, Juul A, Lanng S, et al: Diminished concentrations of insulin-like growth factor I in cystic fibrosis. Arch Dis Child 1995;72:494–497.

12 Machogu E, Cao Y, Miller T, Simpson P, Levy H, Quintero D, Goday PS: Comparison of WHO and CDC growth charts in predicting pulmonary outcomes in cystic fibrosis. J Pediatr Gastroenterol Nutr 2015;60:378–383.

13 Lahiri T, Hempstead SE, Brady C, et al: Clinical practice guidelines from the cystic fibrosis foundation for preschoolers with cystic fibrosis. Pediatrics 2016; 137:pii:e20151784.

14 Turck D, Braegger CP, Colombo C, et al: ESPEN-ESPGHAN-ECFS guidelines on nutrition care for infants, children, and adults with cystic fibrosis. Clin Nutr 2016;35:557–577.

15 Sanders DB, Li Z, Laxova A, Rock MJ, et al: Risk factors for the progression of cystic fibrosis lung disease throughout childhood. Ann Am Thorac Soc 2014; 11:63–72.

16 Lebwohl B, Sanders DS, Green PHR: Coeliac disease. Lancet 2017;28:pii:S0140-6736(17)31796-8.

17 Mora S: Celiac disease in children: impact on bone health. Rev Endocr Metab Disord 2008;9:123–130.

18 Bianchi ML, Bardella MT: Bone in celiac disease. Osteoporos Int 2008;19:1705–1716.

19 Kuehn BM: Food allergies becoming more common. JAMA 2008;300.2358.

20 Christie L, Hine RJ, Parker JG, et al: Food allergies in children affect nutrient intake and growth. J Am Diet Assoc 2002;102:1648–1651.

21 Robbins KA, Wood RA, Keet CA: Milk allergy is associated with decreased growth in US children. J Allergy Clin Immunol 2014;134:1466–1468.e6.

22 Flammarion S, Santos C, Guimber D, et al: Diet and nutritional status of children with food allergies. Pediatr Allergy Immunol 2011;22:161–165.

23 Thapar A, Cooper M: Attention deficit hyperactivity disorder. Lancet 2016;387:1240–1250.

24 Takeda S, Karsenty G: Molecular bases of the sympathetic regulation of bone mass. Bone 2008;42:837–840.

25 Wren TA, Kalkwarf HJ, Zemel BS, et al; Bone Mineral Density in Childhood Study Group: Longitudinal tracking of dual-energy X-ray absorptiometry bone measures over 6 years in children and adolescents: persistence of low bone mass to maturity. J Pediatr 2014;164:1280–1285.e2.

26 Groenman AP, Schweren LJ, Dietrich A, Hoekstra PJ: An update on the safety of psychostimulants for the treatment of attention-deficit/hyperactivity disorder. Expert Opin Drug Saf 2017;16:455–464.

Koletzko B, Shamir R, Turck D, Phillip M (eds): Nutrition and Growth: Yearbook 2018.
World Rev Nutr Diet. Basel, Karger, 2018, vol 117, pp 111–128 (DOI: 10.1159/000484502)

Early Nutrition and Its Effect on Growth, Body Composition and Later Obesity

Kamilla G. Eriksen · Mads V. Lind · Anni Larnkjær · Christian Mølgaard · Kim F. Michaelsen

Department of Nutrition, Exercise and Sports, University of Copenhagen, Copenhagen, Denmark

Adequate nutrition in the first 2 years of life is essential for both short- and long-term health. Malnutrition in the early years of life increases the risk of later chronic diseases. There is a wealth of studies available within this area of research, and this chapter specifically looks at growth and body composition as outcome measures in countries where obesity and related diseases in later life is a large public health problem.

For this short review, we have included 10 publications on the topic of early nutrition and its effect on growth, body composition, and later obesity. We think these 10 included publications, published during the period of July 1, 2016 to June 30, 2017, are of special interest and all present findings can shape future research on this topic. We have chosen to focus on 3 key areas in this review; (i) human milk composition, including studies on breast milk minerals, hormones, and free amino acids (FAA) concentrations (4 studies), (ii) protein intake and later growth, including studies on how protein intake in early childhood is associated with body mass index (BMI; 4 studies), and lastly (iii) early infant feeding and later overweight and obesity, including studies on infant breastfeeding and circadian feeding pattern and the association with later overweight and obesity (2 studies).

Key articles reviewed for this chapter

Human Milk Composition

Associations between human breast milk hormones and adipocytokines and infant growth and body composition in the first 6 months of life

Fields DA, George B, Williams M, Whitaker K, Allison DB, Teague A, Demerath EW

Pediatr Obes Pediatr Obes 2017;12(suppl 1):78–85

Higher leptin but not human milk macronutrient concentration distinguishes normal-weight from obese mothers at 1-month postpartum

De Luca A, Frasquet-Darrieux M, Gaud M-A, Christin P, Boquien C-Y, Millet C, Herviou M, Darmaun D, Robins RJ, Ingrand P, Hankard R

PLoS One 2016;11:e0168568

Free amino acids in human milk and associations with maternal anthropometry and infant growth

Larnkjær A, Bruun S, Pedersen D, Zachariassen G, Barkholt V, Agostoni C, Mølgaard C, Husby S, Michaelsen KF

J Pediatr Gastroenterol Nutr 2016;63:374–378

Minerals and trace elements in human breast milk are associated with Guatemalan infant anthropometric outcomes within the first 6 months

Li C, Solomons NW, Scott ME, Koski KG

J Nutr 2016;146:2067–2074

Protein Intake and Later Growth

Protein intake and dietary glycemic load of 4-year-olds and association with adiposity and serum insulin at 7 years of age: sex-nutrient and nutrient-nutrient interactions

Durão C, Oliveira A, Santos AC, Severo M, Guerra A, Barros H, Lopes C

Int J Obes (Lond) 2017;41:533–541

Dietary intake of protein in early childhood is associated with growth trajectories between 1 and 9 years of age

Braun KV, Erler NS, Kiefte-de Jong JC, Jaddoe VW, van den Hooven EH, Franco OH, Voortman T

J Nutr 2016;146:2361–2367

The association of trajectories of protein intake and age-specific protein intakes from 2 to 22 years with BMI in early adulthood

Wright M, Sotres-Alvarez D, Mendez MA, Adair L

Br J Nutr 2017;117:750–758

Early life protein intake: food sources, correlates, and tracking across the first 5 years of life

Campbell KJ, Abbott G, Zheng M, McNaughton SA

J Acad Nutr Diet 2017;117:1188–1197

Human Milk Composition

Associations between human breast milk hormones and adipocytokines and infant growth and body composition in the first 6 months of life

Fields DA[1], George B[2,3], Williams M[4], Whitaker K[5], Allison DB[2,3], Teague A[1], Demerath EW[4]

[1]Department of Pediatrics, University of Oklahoma Health Sciences Center and CMRI Metabolic Research Program, Oklahoma City, OK, USA; [2]Department of Biostatistics, University of Alabama at Birmingham, Birmingham, AL, USA; [3]Nutrition Obesity Research Center, Birmingham, AL, USA; [4]Department of Obstetrics and Gynecology, Division of Maternal Fetal Medicine, University of Oklahoma Health Sciences Center, Oklahoma City, OK, USA; [5]Division of Epidemiology and Community Health, University of Minnesota School of Public Health, Minneapolis, MN, USA

Pediatr Obes 2017;12(suppl 1):78–85

Background: The concentration of hormones in human breast milk (HBM) and the association with infant growth and body composition needs investigation.
Objectives: In this study, the relationship between the HBM content of insulin, glucose, leptin, interleukin-6 and tumor necrosis factor-α and the maternal BMI, lactation stage (month 1 vs. 6), offspring sex and body composition was explored.
Methods: HBM was collected from 37 exclusively breastfeeding mothers at 1 and 6 months of lactation and analyzed for concentration of various hormones. The maternal BMI ranged from 19 to 47. The infants (16 girls, 21 boys) had body composition measured using dual-energy X-ray absorptiometry.
Results: There was an effect modification by infant sex and maternal BMI on the insulin levels in HBM ($p = 0.032$) such that insulin was 229% higher in obese mothers nursing female infants than in normal-weight mothers nursing female infants and 179% higher than obese mothers nursing male infants.

For leptin, a positive association with BMI category was observed ($p < 0.0001$), such that overweight and obese mothers had 96.5 and 315.1% higher leptin levels than normal-weight mothers, respectively. Leptin decreased 33.7% from 1 to 6 months, controlling for maternal BMI category and sex ($p = 0.0004$). Furthermore, the month 1 leptin concentrations were inversely associated with infant length ($p = 0.026$), percent body fat ($p = 0.022$), total fat mass ($p = 0.023$), and trunk fat mass ($p = 0.011$) at 6 months. No associations or modifications were observed for glucose, tumor necrosis factor-α or interleukin-6.

Conclusion: These data indicate that HBM is modified by maternal adiposity, infant sex, and stage of lactation regarding the concentration of insulin and leptin and that these might influence infant growth and body composition.

Comments on this manuscript will be together with comments on the next manuscript.

Higher leptin but not human milk macronutrient concentration distinguishes normal-weight from obese mothers at 1-month postpartum

De Luca A[1, 2], Frasquet-Darrieux M[3, 4], Gaud M-A[3–5], Christin P[5, 6], Boquien C-Y[7, 8], Millet C[9], Herviou M[3, 4], Darmaun D[7, 8], Robins RJ[10], Ingrand P[3, 4], Hankard R[1, 11]

[1]INSERM U 1069, Tours, France; [2]University Hospital of Tours, Tours, France; [3]INSERM CIC 1402, Poitiers, France; [4]University of Poitiers, Poitiers, France; [5]Pediatrics-Child Nutrition, University Hospital of Poitiers, Poitiers, France; [6]Maternity, General Hospital of Chatellerault, Chatellerault, France; [7]INRA UMR 1280, Institut des Maladies de l'Appareil Digestif, University Hospital of Nantes, Nantes, France; [8]Centre de Recherche en Nutrition Humaine Ouest, Nantes, France; [9]Nuclear Medicine Laboratory, University Hospital of Poitiers, Poitiers, France; [10]Elucidation of Biosynthesis by Isotopic Spectrometry Group, CEISAM, CNRS-University of Nantes UMR 6230, Nantes, France; [11]University F Rabelais, Tours, France

PLoS One 2016;11:e0168568

Background: It has been shown that the weight gain during the first month of life of exclusively breastfed infants born to obese mothers is less compared to infants of normal-weight mothers. Our hypothesis is that human milk composition and volume may differ between obese and normal-weight mothers.

Objectives: To investigate the difference in human milk from exclusively breastfeeding obese and normal-weight mothers regarding milk leptin and macronutrient concentrations and volume at 1 month postpartum. The maternal and infant characteristics for the 2 groups were compared as a secondary aim.

Methods: In this cross-sectional observational study, 50 obese mothers and 50 normal-weight mothers were matched regarding age, parity, ethnic origin, and educational level. All mothers exclusively breastfed their infants for at least 1 month. Human milk samples were collected at an early lactation stage (1 month postpartum) and the volume was assessed. Physical examinations of the mother and infant were conducted at 1 month postpartum.

Results: Human milk from obese, exclusively breastfeeding mothers showed a higher leptin concentration compared to normal-weight, exclusively breastfeeding mothers (4.8 ± 2.7 vs. 2.5 ± 1.5 ng/mL, $p < 0.001$). No difference was observed regarding the concentration of protein, lipid, and carbohydrate and milk volume between obese and normal-weight mothers. Likewise, the infant weight gain during for the first month of life was the same for the 2 groups.

Conclusion: The breast milk of obese and normal-weight mothers differed regarding the leptin concentration with higher concentrations in the milk of obese mothers. However, there was no difference in the macronutrient concentration or in infant growth up to 1 month postpartum. The influence on later growth of the higher leptin content remains to be investigated.

Comments The composition of human breast milk is complex and changes according to lactation stages and varies between mothers [1, 2]. The impact of maternal factors on the human milk composition has attained considerable interest, especially the impact of maternal adiposity due to the growing number of overweight and obese mothers in many parts of the world. In the 2 studies by Fields et al. [3] and De Luca et al. [4], the influence of maternal BMI on leptin concentrations at 1 month postpartum and growth were investigated and adds interesting knowledge to this topic. Both studies found that leptin concentration in breast milk was positively associated with maternal BMI. In the study by Fields et al. [3], insulin was also measured and an interesting interaction between maternal BMI and infant sex was observed, indicating differential sex-based composition of breast milk. A modifying effect on breast milk composition has also been reported for macronutrients and volume [5, 6], which support that a sex-dimorphism in breast milk could be present. A limitation of the present study is the small sample size, and future studies based on larger sample size are warranted to further investigate this remarkable potential sex differences and the mechanism behind.

De Luca et al. [4] did not find a lower weight gain in infants born to obese mothers during the first month of life compared to infants born to normal-weight mothers. The hypothesis suggested by De Luca et al. [4] regarding an association between leptin in breast milk and weight gain during the first month was thus not supported. In the study by De Luca et al. [4], there was no follow-up with later growth measurements, but in the study by Fields et al. [3] growth and body composition up to 6 months of age were determined. Here breast milk leptin concentrations at 1 month postpartum were inversely associated with length and adiposity measures at 6 months postpartum and tended to be negatively associated with weight gain. These are new interesting findings, and existing studies show conflicting results [7, 8]. Studies looking at the role of leptin and other low-abundant proteins in human breast milk in relation to both maternal factors and infant outcomes, such as growth and body composition, are emerging and warranted. Breastfeeding is still advisable for all women, and as pre-pregnancy obesity is a growing public health concern, this area of research is of immediate importance.

Free amino acids in human milk and associations with maternal anthropometry and infant growth

Larnkjær A[1], Bruun S[2], Pedersen D[1], Zachariassen G[2], Barkholt V[3], Agostoni C[4], Mølgaard C[1, 2], Husby S[2], Michaelsen KF[1]

[1]Department of Nutrition, Exercise and Sports, Faculty of Science, University of Copenhagen, Copenhagen, Denmark; [2]Hans Christian Andersen Children's Hospital, Odense University Hospital, Odense, Demark; [3]Department of Systems Biology, Technical University of Denmark, Lyngby, Denmark; [4]Pediatric Clinic, IRCCS Ospedale Maggiore Policlinico, University of Milan, Milan, Italy

J Pediatr Gastroenterol Nutr 2016;63:374–378

Background: The concentrations of free amino acids (FAA); glutamic acid and glutamine, are high in breast milk, and studies with infant formula have suggested that FAA, especially glutamic acid, can affect appetite and thus downregulate dietary intake.

Objectives: The objective of this study was to investigate: (i) the association between glutamic acid or glutamine concentrations in breast milk and current size or early infant growth in fully breastfed Danish infants (using growth as a proxy for breast milk intake) and (ii) how maternal anthropometry was associated with these FFA concentrations in breast milk.

Methods: From a subgroup of 78 mother-infant pairs, of which 50 infants were fully breastfeed, from the Odense Child Cohort, breast milk samples, infant feeding practice data and infant weight and length were collected at 4 months postpartum. The FAA was analyzed by reverse-phase high-performance liquid chromatography.

Results: There was no correlation between the 2 FAA and infant weight or BMI. Infant length at 4 months of age was, however, positively associated with glutamine ($p = 0.013$), but the correlation was attenuated when controlled for birth length ($p = 0.089$). There was a large variation in the concentration of the FAA between mothers. Glutamic acid was positively correlated with mother's pre-pregnancy weight and height ($p \leq 0.028$), but not BMI.

Conclusion: The hypothesis that a high content of glutamic acid and glutamine in breast milk can downregulate milk intake to a degree affecting early growth could not be confirmed in this study. Maternal factors associated with the concentrations of these FAA in milk and the potential influence on the infant should be investigated further.

Comments In this study by Larnkjær et al. [9], the hypothesis that high breast milk glutamic acid and glutamine concentrations downregulate milk intake to a degree that affects infant growth could not be confirmed. However, this study did not measure breast milk intake, but used infant growth as a proxy measure of intake, and furthermore the sample size was small ($n = 78$). No other study has yet investigated the association between milk glutamic acid and glutamine concentrations and infant breast milk intake, which is needed to either reject or accept the hypothesis. The data available in this area of research has been taken from formula-fed infants given hydrolyzed formula that has a high concentration of FAA and nitrogen. These studies have shown a lower intake of the hydrolyzed formula and a growth pattern closer to the pattern of breastfed infants [10, 11]. Furthermore, an intervention study found that adding free glutamic acid to infant formula resulted in a significant reduction in formula intake compared to ordinary formula [12]. This current study by Larnkjær et al. [9] also investigated maternal determinants of breast milk FAA concentrations and found that maternal weight and height were positively associated with the concentration of free glutamic acid in breast milk. An increase in maternal weight of 1 kg corresponded to an increase of 5.6 µmol/L glutamic acid concentration. This has not previously been investigated by others, suggesting the need for further research in maternal determinants of milk FAA concentrations.

Minerals and trace elements in human breast milk are associated with Guatemalan infant anthropometric outcomes within the first 6 months

Li C[1], Solomons NW[4], Scott ME[2, 3], Koski KG[1, 3]

[1]School of Dietetics and Human Nutrition, [2]Institute of Parasitology, and [3]Centre for Host-Parasite Interactions, McGill University, Montreal, Canada; [4]Center for Studies of Sensory Impairment, Aging, and Metabolism (CeSSIAM), Guatemala City, Guatemala

J Nutr 2016;146:2067–2074

Background: Infants are relying on breast milk as the only source of nutrients in the first few months of life, but it is not known how breast milk mineral and trace elements are associated with infant growth.

Objectives: To investigate the concentration of Guatemalan mothers' breast milk mineral and trace element concentrations at three lactation stages to estimate the total daily infant intakes and to determine whether infant intakes were associated with early infant growth.

Methods: In this cross-sectional study, breast milk samples were collected from Mam-Mayan mothers during transitional (5–17 days, $n = 56$), early (18–46 days, $n = 75$), and established lactation (4–6 months, $n = 103$) via full manual expression. Infant z-scores for weight (WAZ), length (LAZ), and head circumference (HCAZ) were measured from exclusively or predominantly breast-fed infants. Inductively coupled plasma-mass spectrometry was used to analyze calcium, potassium, magnesium, sodium, copper, iron, manganese, rubidium, selenium, strontium, and zinc concentrations. Daily breast milk mineral intakes were based on estimations. Principal component analyses identified clusters of minerals; principal components (PCs) were used in multiple linear regression analyses for anthropometric outcomes.

Results: Guatemalan infants had a high rate of growth faltering in this study, with 45% stunting at 4–6 months of age. Estimated infant intakes of calcium, magnesium, potassium, sodium, and selenium were below the Institute of Medicine Adequate Intake for males and females at all 3 stages of lactation. In early lactation, PC1 (calcium, magnesium, potassium, rubidium, and strontium intakes) was positively associated with infant WAZ, LAZ, and HCAZ. In established lactation, the same PC with sodium added was positively associated with all 3 anthropometric outcomes; a second PC (PC2: zinc, copper, and selenium intakes) was associated with WAZ and LAZ but not HCAZ.

Conclusion: A higher intake of breast milk minerals and trace elements of Guatemalan infants could be beneficial for infant growth during early infancy.

Comments The investigation of breast milk micronutrient composition has started to emerge in the scientific literature, especially because reliable quantification methods have evolved over the past few years [13]. However limited studies are available in this area of research. For instance, few high-quality studies are available on how maternal micronutrient deficiencies influence breast milk micronutrient composition. More importantly for breast milk minerals, the adequate concentration of micronutrients in human milk for healthy growth and development are unknown. Furthermore, very limited evidence is available on how breast milk micronutrient composition is associated with infant growth. This study by Li et al. [14] contributes to the knowledge regarding how breast milk mineral and trace element concentrations are associated with infant growth in a population in Guatemala where infant growth faltering is common, and where maternal height is one of the lowest in the world [15]. However, there are several limitations to the results and conclusions by Li et al. [14]. In this study, breast milk intakes were not measured but based on estimates. This is a limitation as breast milk intake often varies substantially among exclusively breastfed infants [16], and it is therefore not possible to distinguish if the observed association with growth reported by Li et al. [14] is driven by infant breast milk intakes or by breast milk mineral concentrations. Another general limitation is that, it is not possible to determine if the breast milk mineral concentrations reported in this study are *too* low or inadequate for healthy growth and development, as it is not yet known what the adequate micronutrient concentrations in breast milk are. Concluding on any inadequacy of breast milk micronutrient concentrations should thus be done with caution, especially if neither maternal nor infant status are investigated. This study by Li et al. [14] highlights the need for further research on breast milk micronutrient composition in resource-poor settings where growth faltering is experienced in early infancy during the period of exclusive breastfeeding and the need for establishing reference values in populations with adequate nutritional status.

Protein Intake and Later Growth

Protein intake and dietary glycemic load of 4-year-olds and association with adiposity and serum insulin at 7 years of age: sex-nutrient and nutrient-nutrient interactions

Durão C[1], Oliveira A[1, 2], Santos AC[1, 2], Severo M[1, 2], Guerra A[3], Barros H[1, 2], Lopes C[1, 2]

[1]EPIUnit – Institute of Public Health, Universidade do Porto, Porto, Portugal; [2]Department of Clinical Epidemiology, Predictive Medicine and Public Health, University of Porto Medical School, Universidade do Porto, Porto, Portugal; [3]Department of Pediatrics, University of Porto Medical School, Universidade do Porto, Porto, Portugal

Int J Obes (Lond) 2017;41:533–541

Background: Limited prospective studies have investigated the role of protein intake (PI) and dietary glycemic load (GL) in preschool children on later adiposity.

Objective: The aim of this study was to examine the association of PI and GL at 4 years with adiposity and fasting serum insulin (FSI) at 7 years, and to evaluate if sex modified this association. Furthermore, a possible interaction between PI and GL was examined.

Methods: For the analyses in this study, the population-based birth cohort, Generation XXI (Porto, Portugal, 2005–2006) including 1999 singleton children was used. A 3-day food diary was used to assess the diet at 4 years of age. Both PI and GL (g/day) were energy-adjusted and converted into sex-specific tertiles (T). World Health Organization (WHO) standards were used to calculate the BMI z-scores at 7 years of age. Body composition was determined by bioelectric impedance and sex-specific z-scores were computed for fat mass index (FMI), waist-to-height ratio (W/Ht), and FSI. Linear regression was used to estimate associations.

Results: PI in girls and boys were similar while girls had slightly lower GL than boys. For both girls and boys, PI was positively associated with BMI (T2 vs. T1: $\beta = 0.187$; 95% CI 0.015–0.359) and (T3 vs. T1: $\beta = 0.205$; 95% CI 0.003–0.406, respectively), while PI was only associated with FSI in boys (T3 vs. T1: $\beta = 0.207$; 95% CI 0.011–0.404; P-interaction = 0.026). Similarly GL was associated with BMI only in boys (T3 vs. T1: $\beta = 0.362$; 95% CI 0.031–0.693; P-interaction = 0.006). Significant interactions between PI and GL were found on the association with FMI ($p = 0.019$) and W/Ht ($p = 0.039$) in boys only. Boys belonging to the third tertile of both PI and GL at 4 years had higher FMI ($\beta = 0.505$; 95% CI 0.085–0.925) and W/Ht ($\beta = 0.428$; 95% CI 0.022–0.834) 3 years later.

Conclusion: This study showed that for preschool children PI was positively associated with later BMI in both sexes, while PI was positively associated with FSI in boys only. Dietary GL was only positively associated with adiposity in boys.

Comments This study is one of few studies evaluating the effect of higher PI on later obesity in preschool-aged children. The study showed, like several other studies with children in different age groups, that high PI was associated with higher BMI years later in both girls and boys [17]. Furthermore, the study focused on sex differences in response to nutrients and showed some interesting results. PI was positively associated with serum insulin and dietary GL to BMI in boys only. In girls, the influence of energy intake was independent of macronutrient distribution, while in contrast, boys were dependent on energy from either protein or carbohydrate. The authors discussed possible mechanism behind this sex differences in response to the same food. They proposed that physiologically females prefer to use fat as a substrate while males have a larger propensity to rely on glucose and protein metabolism. Another interesting topic in this study was the analyses of possible nutrient-nutrient interactions. The study showed that dietary GL interacts with PI in boys. Boys in the highest tertile of both GL and PI at 4 years had higher FMI and waist/height ratio at 7 years of age. Possible mechanisms behind this association to central adiposity were also discussed. High PI may increase levels of branched-chain amino acids, which stimulate secretion of IGF-1 and insulin. Glucose similarly stimulate insulin production, and it is known that males are more sensitive to insulin and thereby develop central adiposity. However, the authors underline that more studies are needed to further understand the sex-nutrient and nutrient-nutrient interactions.

Dietary intake of protein in early childhood is associated with growth trajectories between 1 and 9 years of age

Braun KV[1, 2], Erler NS[2, 3], Kiefte-de Jong JC[2, 5], Jaddoe VW[1, 2, 4], van den Hooven EH[2], Franco OH[2], Voortman T[1, 2]

[1]The Generation R Study Group and [2]Departments of Epidemiology, [3]Biostatistics, and [7]Paediatrics, Erasmus MC, University Medical Center, Rotterdam, Netherlands; [5]Leiden University College, The Hague, Netherlands

J Nutr 2016;146:2361–2367

Background: High protein intake in infancy may lead to a higher BMI in childhood. However, it is not known whether different sources of protein have the same relation to later BMI.

Objective: Associations between intake of total protein, different protein sources, and single amino acids in early childhood and later height, weight, and BMI up to the age of 9 years were analyzed.

Methods: The children analyzed ($n = 3,564$) participated in multi-ethnic population-based prospective cohort study, the Generation R, in Rotterdam, The Netherlands. A food-frequency questionnaire was used to asses intakes of total protein, animal protein, vegetable protein, and individual amino acids (including methionine, arginine, lysine, threonine, valine, leucine, isoleucine, phenylalanine, tryptophan, histidine, cysteine, tyrosine, alanine, asparagine, glutamine, glycine, proline, and serine) at 1 year. At the approximate ages of 14, 18, 24, 30, 36, and 45 months and at 6 and 9 years, height and weight were measured and BMI calculated.

Results: Linear mixed models were used for analyses and after adjustment for confounders, a 10-g higher total protein intake/day at 1 year was significantly associated with a 0.03-SD greater height (95% CI 0.00–0.06), a 0.06-SD higher weight (95% CI 0.03–0.09), and a 0.05-SD higher BMI (95% CI 0.03–0.08) up to the age of 9 years. Animal protein intake was more strongly associated with BMI than vegetable protein intake, but dairy and non-dairy animal protein did not differ. Similarly, there were no differences between specific amino acids. There were no significant interactions between protein intake and age or outcome measurements, sex or ethnicity.

Conclusion: Higher intake of protein at 1 year of age, especially animal protein, was associated with a greater height, weight, and BMI in childhood up to 9 year of age. The association was not different for dairy and non-dairy animal protein. However, the role of growth hormones and whether protein intake in early childhood affects health later in life need further investigation.

Comments	This study is one of several studies based on data from the Generation R study [20]. It is interesting both because of the large sample size followed by longitudinal anthropometric measurements up to the age of 9 years. Furthermore, this study is interesting as it investigates the impact of different protein sources. The basis for this is the detailed analyses of the food intake by using a semi-quantitative FFQ with 211 food items, which estimates intake of total protein, animal protein, and vegetable protein. Furthermore, the intake of animal protein was divided into dairy and non-dairy protein, and the intake of different amino acids were calculated. The FFQ was validated against three 24-h-recalls. The detailed food registration provides an opportunity to investigate which role different proteins and amino acids have for growth and the risk of development of later overweight or obesity.
	The study also underlines that the positive association with height, weight, and BMI is stronger for animal protein intake than vegetable protein. Studies have further shown that there is a difference in the effect of dairy and non-dairy animal protein; a high intake of milk, but not meat, increases IGF-1 and insulin in short-term studies with school-aged boys [21, 22]. It was thus surprising that Braun et al. [19] did not find any differences between diary and non-dairy animal protein. The idea suggested by others concerning a special growth stimulating effect of certain amino acids like arginine and lysine was however not confirmed in this study. More studies are needed to understand the effect of different protein sources.

The association of trajectories of protein intake and age-specific protein intakes from 2 to 22 years with BMI in early adulthood

Wright M[1], Sotres-Alvarez D[2], Mendez MA[1], Adair L[1]

[1]Department of Nutrition, University of North Carolina at Chapel Hill, Chapel Hill, NC, USA;
[2]Department of Biostatistics, University of North Carolina at Chapel Hill, Chapel Hill, NC, USA

Br J Nutr 2017;117:750–758

The early protein hypothesis has been examined in multiple cohorts; however, protein intake measured at multiple time-points from early childhood to young adulthood has not been assessed. This study associates the intake across childhood, adolescent, and young adulthood to adult BMI. The association of estimated protein intake at 2, 11, 15, 19, and 22 years were assessed with age- and sex-standardized BMI at 22 years (early adulthood). Linear regression models with dietary and anthropometric data from a Filipino birth cohort (1985–2005, n = 2,586) were used to associate protein intake and adult BMI. Latent growth curve analysis was used to identify trajectories of protein intake relative to age-specific recommended daily allowance (intake in g/kg body weight) from 2 to 22 years. This resulted in four mutually exclusive trajectories of protein intake, which were related to early adulthood BMI using linear regression models. Lean mass and fat mass were determined by skinfold measurements, which were secondary outcomes. Regression models adjusted for several socioeconomic, dietary, and anthropometric confounders from early life and adulthood were used. It was found that a higher protein intake relative to needs at age 2 years was positively associated with BMI and lean mass at age 22 years, in females but not males. Protein intakes at ages 11, 15, and 22 years were overall inversely associated with early adulthood BMI, fat, and fat-free mass in both males and females, however, the associations were more consistent in females. Individuals were then classified into four mutually exclusive trajectories: (i) normal consumers, who had a protein intake just above recommendations (referent trajectory, 58% of cohort), (ii) high protein consumers in infancy, with a subsequent protein intake just above recommendations (20%), (iii) usually high consumers who had high intakes before age 19, with very high intake at age 11 (18%), and (iv) always high consumers, who had high protein intake at 2 years of age and thereafter (5%). Compared with the normal consumers "usually high," consumption was inversely associated with BMI, lean mass, and fat mass at age 22 years whereas "always high" consumption was inversely associated with lean mass in males only. It seemed that protein intake more close to adulthood was a more important contributor to early adult BMI relative to early-childhood protein intake; protein intake trajectory history was differentially associated with adulthood body sizes.

Comments on this manuscript will be together with comments on the next manuscript.

Early life protein intake: food sources, correlates, and tracking across the first 5 years of life

Campbell KJ, Abbott G, Zheng M, McNaughton SA

Institute for Physical Activity and Nutrition, School of Excecise and Nutrition Sciences, Deakin University, Geelong, Victoria, Australia

J Acad Nutr Diet 2017;117:1188–1197

Background: A high consumption of protein has been associated with accelerated growth and adiposity in early childhood.

Objective: The aim of this study was to describe dietary intake, food sources, correlates, and tracking of protein intake in young children.

Methods: This study was a secondary analysis of the Melbourne Infant Feeding Activity and Nutrition Trial which consisted of first-time mothers and their child (n = 542). They participated in an 18-month intervention to prevent childhood obesity, and the cohort was followed-up with no intervention when children were aged 3.5 and 5 years. Dietary data were collected using three 24-h dietary recalls at ages 9 and 18 months as well as 3.5 and 5 years. Protein intake, food sources, correlates, and tracking of protein were included in the analysis of the main outcomes.

Statistical analyses performed: The child and maternal correlates of protein intake were identified using linear regression models and tracking of protein intake was examined using Pearson correlations of residualized protein scores between time points.

Results: The mean protein (g/day) intake was 29.7 ± 11.0, 46.3 ± 11.5, 54.2 ± 13.8, and 60.0 ± 14.8 at 9 and 18 months at 3.5 and 5 years, respectively. The mean protein intake at all age groups was

2–3 times greater than age-appropriate Australian recommendations. The primary source of protein at 9 months was breast/formula milk. At later ages, the principal sources were milk/milk products, breads/cereals, and meat/meat products. Significant predictors of high protein intake at different time-points were earlier breastfeeding cessation, earlier introduction of solids, high dairy milk consumption (≥500 mL), and high maternal education ($p < 0.05$). A slight tracking for protein intakes were found at 9 months, 18 months, and 5 years of age ($r = 0.16$–0.21; $p < 0.01$).

Conclusion: This study provides insights into the food sources of young children's high protein intakes, and confirms that early life protein intake tracks slightly up to the age of 5 years. Furthermore, this study found correlates of protein intake that might be relevant for future interventions. The findings of the present study have the potential to provide information for nutritional intervention studies to target high protein intake as a potential way to mitigate later obesity risk at an early age.

Comments   The early protein hypothesis state that high protein intake early in life may increase the risk of obesity later in life. This is being extensively researched and the 2 present studies, each contribute by (i) examining the association between early life protein intake and BMI/adiposity in adulthood and (ii) examining food sources of protein and early determinants of protein intake.

In the first study, Wright et al. [23] did not show strong associations between protein intake and BMI or adiposity. Furthermore, infants with high early life protein intake and subsequent "normal" protein intake were not different from infants with "normal" protein intake throughout infancy, childhood, and adolescent. However, the study reported sex-specific associations with protein intake, which is in line with other studies showing that the associations between protein intake and BMI/adiposity tends to be stronger in girls than in boys [24]. There might be several reasons why the associations between protein intake and BMI was not as strong in this study as indicated in previous studies. First, the present study measured protein intake throughout childhood, adolescent, and early adulthood, something that has not often been done. The use of repeated dietary assessment is important when examining long-term outcomes, and adds value to the results. However, a limitation of the study is that protein intake was not measured as early as other studies, which have shown a strong association between 1 year protein intake and later adiposity [20]. Furthermore, multiple assessments of diet throughout infancy would add valuable knowledge in determining potential critical phases of exposure. A strength of this study is the long follow-up and measurement of BMI and adiposity in adulthood. However, the results did not show clear differences in lean versus fat mass accretion as the association estimates were of the same direction – therefore, future studies need to add more accurate adiposity measurements. Finally, the study cohort was different compared to other cohorts examining early life protein intake and adiposity, as it had a high prevalence of infant undernutrition and the infant diet had a high grain content and was low in animal protein. In addition, the cohort had a low intake of dairy protein (<10% of protein intake) compared to other cohorts (40–80% of protein intake). This is of special interest because dairy protein has been linked to a specific amino acid composition and thus hypothesized to be more pro-obesogenic/growth spurting, especially in infancy/early childhood compared to other protein sources [17]. Thus, it could be speculated that the lack of high dairy protein intake in infancy contributed to the low effect estimates on later adiposity.

Multiple aspects of the early protein hypothesis remain to be investigated and the findings from Wright et al. [23] warrants further investigation, preferably randomized intervention trials. For such trials, it is important to know which components to target for intervention. The study by Campbell et al. [25] provided information on the major food sources and other determinants of early life protein intake. The authors showed that milk, cereals, and meat were the main contributors of protein intake at age 9 months to 5 years. The protein intake was substantially higher than the recommendations, which gives room for potential interventions. The authors also examined other determinants of high protein intake to identify potential targets for interventions and found that early introduction of solid foods, early cessation of breastfeeding, and high milk consumption was associated with higher protein intake. Protein intake was weakly correlated (Pearson's correlation in the order of 0.16–0.21) across different timepoints in infancy indicating tracking.

The present study by Campbell et al. [25] is in line with other findings showing that the intake of dairy and meat products in early life contribute to the majority of the protein intake. Among European populations, dairy consumption contributed the most protein at 6 months, decreasing with age until meat and dairy intake contributed almost equally at 24 months of age [26]. Based on these results targeting these foods, by reducing intake, and thereby lowering protein intake could be suggested as a potential intervention in early childhood. However, good sources of protein are also good sources of other key nutrients such as several vitamins and calcium, as also highlighted by Campbell et al. [25] Thus, potential future interventions regarding diet with reduced protein content should still have sufficient amount of other essential nutrients. Furthermore, careful examination of protein intake based on population-specific intake is necessary as different protein sources might vary in relevance between populations as seen in the Wright et al. [23] and Campbell et al. [25] studies.

One further aspect that is intriguing from the studies of Wright et al. [23], Durão et al. [18] and Braun et al. [19] is at what age the association between protein intake and BMI/body composition switches. While all three studies show associations between high protein intake and adiposity at age 1, 2, and 4 years of age, the study by Wright et al. [23] also show opposite associations at age 11. In adulthood, a higher protein intake has been linked to increased satiety, increased thermogenesis, maintenance or accretion of fat-free mass, and may thus be beneficial for weight loss and weight maintenance [27]. Thus, it seems that there is an age-dependent effect of protein on body composition. At what point this switch happens and what the biological mechanisms behind it is, is still largely unknown, but could have something to do with pre-pubertal changes in sex and growth hormones and insulin sensitivity. However, this warrants further study.

Infant feeding and growth trajectory patterns in childhood and body composition in young adulthood

Rzehak P[1], Oddy WH[2, 3], Mearin ML[5], Grote V[1], Mori TA[4], Szajewska H[6], Shamir R[7], Koletzko S[8], Weber M[1], Beilin LJ[4], Huang RC[3, 4], Koletzko B[1]; WP10 working group of the Early Nutrition Project

[1]Division of Metabolic and Nutritional Medicine, and [8]Division of Gastroenterology and Hepatology, Dr. von Hauner Children's Hospital, Ludwig-Maximilians Universität München, Munich, Germany; [2]Menzies Institute for Medical Research, The University of Tasmania, Hobart, Tasmania, Australia; [3]Telethon Kids Institute and [4]School of Medicine and Pharmacology, University of Western Australia, Perth, Western Australia, Australia; [5]Department of Paediatrics, Leiden University Medical Center, Leiden, Netherlands; [6]Department of Paediatrics, Medical University of Warsaw, Warsaw, Poland; [7]Institute of Gastroenterology, Nutrition and Liver Disease, Schneider Children's Medical Center, Sackler Faculty of Medicine, Tel Aviv University, Tel Aviv, Israel

Am J Clin Nutr 2017;106:568–580

Background: Growth patterns of breastfed and formula-fed infants differ, with formula-fed infants growing more rapidly than breastfed infants into childhood and adulthood.

Objective: The objectives of this study were to: (i) identify growth patterns and (ii) investigate early nutritional programming potential on growth patterns at 6 years and on body composition at 20 years.

Methods: Data from the West Australian Pregnancy Cohort (Raine) Study and three European cohort studies (European Childhood Obesity Trial, Norwegian Human Milk Study, and Prevention of Coeliac Disease) were combined, harmonized, and pooled to include information on breastfeeding, anthropometry, and body composition. From zero to 6 years, semi-annual anthropometric measurements were available and BMI was calculated. Latent growth mixture modeling was applied to identify growth patterns among the 6,708 individual growth trajectories. The association of full breastfeeding for <3 months compared with ≥3 months with the identified trajectory classes was assessed by logistic regression. Differences in body composition at 20 years (only in the Raine study; based on skinfolds and dual-energy X-ray absorptiometry) among the identified trajectory classes were tested by analysis of variance.

Results: Three BMI trajectory patterns were identified and labeled as follows; class 1: persistent, accelerating, rapid growth (5%); class 2: early, non-persistent, rapid growth (40%); and class 3: normative growth (55%). Full breastfeeding for <3 months was associated with being in rapid-growth class 1 (OR 2.66; 95% CI 1.48–4.79) and class 2 (OR 1.96; 95% CI 1.51–2.55) rather than the normative-growth class 3 after adjustment for covariates. For each additional month of full breastfeeding, there was a reduced risk of being in the rapid growth classes, class 1 and 2 of 17 and 6%, respectively. Both classes showed significant associations with body composition at 20 years ($p < 0.0001$). Children who had a higher probability of being in one of the 2 rapid-trajectory class had higher BMI, skinfolds, and fat mass index at 20 years compared to the normative growth class.

Conclusion: Full breastfeeding for <3 months compared with ≥3 months may be associated with rapid growth in early childhood and body composition in young adulthood. Rapid growth patterns in early childhood could be a mediating link between infant feeding and long-term obesity risk.

Comments   Using growth trajectory pattern analysis, and combining four large cohorts with more than 6,000 participants, the authors were able to distinguish three quite different and interesting growth patterns. The largest group class 3 (normative growth, 55% of the children) had a BMI z-score (BAZ) pattern very close to the WHO growth standards from birth to 6 years. Forty percent of the children had an early non-persistent rapid growth (class 2). The rapid growth started in early infancy and had a mean BAZ of about +1 at 2 years of age. From 2 to 6 years of age, there was a steady decline in BAZ reaching a BAZ of about +0.5 at 6 years of age. The smallest group (5%, persisting, accelerating, rapid growth) had an extreme pattern. BMI only started to increase from the age of about one year and then accelerated steadily until 6 years when it reached about +3 BAZ. A strength of the study is that the Raine cohort was followed to 20 years and it was thus possible to examine the long-term effect of these three distinct growth trajectories on body composition in young adults. As Rzehak et al. [28] underline in their concluding sentence, the results are based on observational data and does not allow conclusions about casual effects of breastfeeding as neither reverse causation nor residual confounding can be ruled out.

It is still discussed if breastfeeding has an effect on the risk of later overweight and obesity. In the Lancet series on breastfeeding from 2016 [29], it was concluded that the evidence was suggestive for a protective effect on breastfeeding. This conclusion was based on a review by Horta et al. [30], which found a risk reduction of 13% based on results from 23 high quality studies. However, in the PROBIT intervention study with a cluster randomized design there was no effect of breastfeeding on later overweight and obesity up to 16 years of age [31]. Apart from residual confounding, reverse causation could also play a role, that is, the weight gain of the infant influences the time when either infant formula or complementary foods are introduced.

Predominantly nighttime feeding and weight outcomes in infants

Cheng TS[1], Loy SL[3, 5], Toh JY[7], Cheung YB[4, 8], Chan JK[2, 3, 5], Godfrey KM[9, 10], Gluckman PD[7, 11], Saw SM[12], Chong YS[7, 13], Lee YS[7, 14], Lek N[1, 5], Chong MF[6, 14], Yap F[1, 5, 15]

Departments of [1]Pediatrics and [2]Reproductive Medicine and [3]KK Research Center, KK Women's and Children's Hospital, Singapore; [4]Center for Quantitative Medicine, [5]Duke-NUS Medical School, Singapore; [6]Clinical Nutrition Research Center, [7]Singapore Institute for Clinical Sciences, Agency for Science, Technology and Research, Singapore; [8]Tampere Center for Child Health Research, University of Tampere and Tampere University Hospital, Tampere, Finland; [9]Medical Research Council Lifecourse Epidemiology Unit, University of Southampton, Southampton, UK; [10]National Institute for Health Research Southampton Biomedical Research Center, University of Southampton and University Hospital Southampton National Health Service Foundation Trust, Southampton, UK; [11]Liggins Institute, University of Auckland, Auckland, New Zealand; [12]Saw Swee Hock School of Public Health and Departments of [13]Obstetrics and Gynaecology and [14]Pediatrics, Yong Loo Lin School of Medicine, National University of Singapore, Singapore; [15]Lee Kong Chian School of Medicine, Nanyang Technological University, Singapore

Am J Clin Nutr 2016;104:380–388

This manuscript is also discussed in Chapter 2, pages 15–38.

Background: The influence of circadian feeding patterns on weight outcomes has been shown in animal and human studies but not in young children. Adults who consume more energy in the evening tend to be overweight or obese, but this has not been examined in infants. Both food and light are important signals influencing biological rhythms.

Objective: The aim of this study was to examine the association of infant circadian feeding patterns at 12 months of age with subsequent growth from 12 to 24 months and weight status at 24 months.

Methods: Mothers from a Singaporean birth cohort ($n = 349$) reported the food given to their infants and the feeding time at 12 months of age. Predominantly daytime (pDT; 07.00–18.59; $n = 282$) and predominantly nighttime (pNT; 19.00–06.59; $n = 67$) feeding infants were defined by whether daytime energy intake was >50 or <50% of total energy intake as assessed with the use of a 24-h dietary recall. These hours were chosen as they are close to sunrise and sunset in Singapore. BMI-for-age z scores (BAZ) were calculated using the WHO Child Growth Standards 2006 to determine changes in BAZ from 12 to 24 months of age and weight status at 24 months of age. Multivariable linear and logistic regression analyses were performed.

Results: Total 24-h energy intake was not different between pNT- and pDT-feeding infants (815 ± 229 compared with 764 ± 222 kcal, respectively; $p = 0.090$). The pNT-feeding infants had a lower percentage of energy from protein compared with the pDT-feeding infants (12.7 ± 2.8 vs. 14.8 ± 3.2%; $p < 0.001$). Compared with pDT feeding, pNT feeding was associated with a higher BAZ gain from 12 to 24 months of age (adjusted β = 0.38; 95% CI 0.11–0.65; $p = 0.006$) and increased risk of overweight at 24 months of age (adjusted OR 2.78; 95% CI 1.11–6.97; $p = 0.029$) after adjusting for maternal age, education, ethnicity, monthly household income, parity, infant BAZ at 12 months of age, feeding mode in the first 6 months of life, and total daily energy intake.

Conclusion: These results suggest that the role of the daily distribution of energy consumption in weight regulation may begin in infancy. A pNT feeding pattern of infants was associated with adiposity gain and risk of overweight in early childhood. The inclusion of advice on the appropriate feeding time may be considered when implementing strategies to combat childhood obesity.

Comments
The effects on growth of many aspects of infant feeding have been examined in detail, for example, breastfeeding versus formula feeding, composition of breast milk, time of introducing complementary foods, and macronutrient intake, and several of these recent studies are included in this chapter and in our chapter in the Nutrition and Growth Yearbook 2017 [1]. This study is interesting because it is the first to examine if circadian infant feeding pattern can influence growth and risk of obesity.

Adults who eat at nighttime have a higher risk of overweight, but most studies have been observational and the mechanisms behind such an effect have not yet been identified [32]. In this study by Cheng et al. [33], the infants who were nighttime feeders (19% of the infants) consumed 63% of their energy between 7 p.m. and 7 a.m., while for the daytime feeders it was only 33%. The largest difference in infant intakes between the 2 groups was from 7 to 10 p.m. A higher proportion of the nighttime feeders were breastfed, both at 6 and 12 months of age, but this was controlled in the analysis of the effect on BMI gain and risk of becoming overweight.

Short sleep duration during infancy has been associated with an increased risk of later overweight [34]. It is possible that there is an interaction between sleep duration and circadian feeding pattern. In the present study, the total sleep duration attenuated the risk of becoming overweight, but the effect was small and sleep duration was only recorded in 41% of the infants.

The mechanisms behind the effect of circadian feeding pattern on BMI seen in this study are unknown and it is not clear to what degree the feeding pattern is driven by the parents or by the infant. Future studies should include measurements of appetite and growth-related hormones, measurements of body composition, and a detailed registration of sleep and food intake. Furthermore, intervention studies could explore the effect of circadian feeding pattern on hormones and other relevant metabolic parameters. Before the mechanisms behind the interesting association found in this study are understood, we will not know if advice on appropriate feeding time will have an effect on growth, later overweight, and obesity.

References

1 Lind MV, Larnkjaer A, Molgaard C, Michaelsen KF: Early nutrition and its effect on growth, body composition, and later obesity. World Rev Nutr Diet 2017;116:118–133.

2 Agostoni C, Carratu B, Boniglia C, Lammardo AM, Riva E, Sanzini E: Free glutamine and glutamic acid increase in human milk through a three-month lactation period. J Pediatr Gastroenterol Nutr 2000;31:508–512.

3 Fields DA, George B, Williams M, Whitaker K, Allison DB, Teague A, et al: Associations between human breast milk hormones and adipocytokines and infant growth and body composition in the first 6 months of life. Pediatr Obes 2017;12(suppl 1):78–85.

4 De Luca A, Frasquet-Darrieux M, Gaud M-A, Christin P, Boquien C-Y, Millet C, et al: Higher leptin but not human milk macronutrient concentration distinguishes normal-weight from obese mothers at 1-month postpartum. PLoS ONE 2016;11:e0168568.

5 Powe CE, Knott CD, Conklin-Brittain N: Infant sex predicts breast milk energy content. Am J Hum Biol 2010;22:50–54.

6 Fujita M, Roth E, Lo YJ, Hurst C, Vollner J, Kendell A: In poor families, mothers' milk is richer for daughters than sons: a test of Trivers-Willard hypothesis in agropastoral settlements in Northern Kenya. Am J Phys Anthropol 2012;149:52–59.

7 Brunner S, Schmid D, Zang K, Much D, Knoeferl B, Kratzsch J, et al: Breast milk leptin and adiponectin in relation to infant body composition up to 2 years. Pediatr Obes 2015;10:67–73.

8 Schuster S, Hechler C, Gebauer C, Kiess W, Kratzsch J: Leptin in maternal serum and breast milk: association with infants' body weight gain in a longitudinal study over 6 months of lactation. Pediatr Res 2011; 70:633–637.

9 Larnkjaer A, Bruun S, Pedersen D, Zachariassen G, Barkholt V, Agostoni C, et al: Free amino acids in human milk and associations with maternal anthropometry and infant growth. J Pediatr Gastroenterol Nutr 2016;63:374–378.

10 Mennella JA, Ventura AK, Beauchamp GK: Differential growth patterns among healthy infants fed protein hydrolysate or cow-milk formulas. Pediatrics 2011;127:110–118.

11 Rzehak P, Sausenthaler S, Koletzko S, Reinhardt D, von Berg A, Kramer U, et al: Short- and long-term effects of feeding hydrolyzed protein infant formulas on growth at ≤6 y of age: results from the German Infant Nutritional Intervention Study. Am J Clin Nutr 2009;89:1846–1856.

12 Ventura AK, Beauchamp GK, Mennella JA: Infant regulation of intake: the effect of free glutamate content in infant formulas. Am J Clin Nutr 2012;95:875–881.

13 Allen LH: Current information gaps in micronutrient research, programs and policy: how can we fill them? World Rev Nutr Diet 2016;115:109–117.

14 Li C, Solomons NW, Scott ME, Koski KG: Minerals and trace elements in human breast milk are associated with guatemalan infant anthropometric outcomes within the first 6 months. J Nutr 2016;146: 2067–2074.

15 NCD Risk Factor Collaboration (NCD-RisC): A century of trends in adult human height. Elife 2016; 5;pii:e13410.

16 Kent JC, Mitoulas LR, Cregan MD, Ramsay DT, Doherty DA, Hartmann PE: Volume and frequency of breastfeedings and fat content of breast milk throughout the day. Pediatrics 2006;117:e387–e395.

17 Weber M, Grote V, Closa-Monasterolo R, Escribano J, Langhendries JP, Dain E, et al: Lower protein content in infant formula reduces BMI and obesity risk at school age: follow-up of a randomized trial. Am J Clin Nutr 2014;99:1041–1051.

18 Durão C, Oliveira A, Santos AC, Severo M, Guerra A, Barros H, et al: Protein intake and dietary glycemic load of 4-year-olds and association with adiposity and serum insulin at 7 years of age: sex-nutrient and nutrient-nutrient interactions. Int J Obes (Lond) 2017;41:533–541.

19 Braun KV, Erler NS, Kiefte-de Jong JC, Jaddoe VW, van den Hooven EH, Franco OH, et al: Dietary intake of protein in early childhood is associated with growth trajectories between 1 and 9 years of age. J Nutr 2016;146:2361–2367.

20 Voortman T, Braun KV, Kiefte-de Jong JC, Jaddoe VW, Franco OH, van den Hooven EH: Protein intake in early childhood and body composition at the age of 6 years: The Generation R Study. Int J Obes (Lond) 2016;40:1018–1025.

21 Hoppe C, Molgaard C, Juul A, Michaelsen KF: High intakes of skimmed milk, but not meat, increase serum IGF-I and IGFBP-3 in eight-year-old boys. Eur J Clin Nutr 2004;58:1211–1216.

22 Hoppe C, Molgaard C, Vaag A, Barkholt V, Michaelsen KF: High intakes of milk, but not meat, increase s-insulin and insulin resistance in 8-year-old boys. Eur J Clin Nutr 2005;59:393–398.

23 Wright M, Sotres-Alvarez D, Mendez MA, Adair L: The association of trajectories of protein intake and age-specific protein intakes from 2 to 22 years with BMI in early adulthood. Br J Nutr 2017;117:750–758.

24 Lind MV, Larnkjaer A, Molgaard C, Michaelsen KF: Dietary protein intake and quality in early life: impact on growth and obesity. Curr Opin Clin Nutr Metab Care 2017;20:71–76.

25 Campbell KJ, Abbott G, Zheng M, McNaughton SA: Early life protein intake: food sources, correlates, and tracking across the first 5 years of life. J Acad Nutr Diet 2017;117:1188–1197.

26 Damianidi L, Gruszfeld D, Verduci E, Vecchi F, Xhonneux A, Langhendries JP, et al: Protein intakes and their nutritional sources during the first 2 years of life: secondary data evaluation from the European Childhood Obesity Project. Eur J Clin Nutr 2016;70: 1291–1297.

27 Paddon-Jones D, Westman E, Mattes RD, Wolfe RR, Astrup A, Westerterp-Plantenga M: Protein, weight management, and satiety. Am J Clin Nutr 2008;87: 1558s–1561s.

28 Rzehak P, Oddy WH, Mearin ML, Grote V, Mori TA, Szajewska H, et al: Infant feeding and growth trajectory patterns in childhood and body composition in young adulthood. Am J Clin Nutr 2017;106:568–580.

29 Victora CG, Bahl R, Barros AJD, França GVA, Horton S, Krasevec J, et al: Breastfeeding in the 21st century: epidemiology, mechanisms, and lifelong effect. Lancet 387:475–490.

30 Horta BL, Loret de Mola C, Victora CG: Long-term consequences of breastfeeding on cholesterol, obesity, systolic blood pressure and type 2 diabetes: a systematic review and meta-analysis. Acta Paediatr 2015;104:30–37.

31 Martin RM, Kramer MS, Patel R, Rifas-Shiman SL, Thompson J, Yang S, et al: Effects of promoting long-term, exclusive breastfeeding on adolescent adiposity, blood pressure, and growth trajectories: a secondary analysis of a randomized clinical trial. JAMA Pediatr 2017;171:e170698.

32 Wang JB, Patterson RE, Ang A, Emond JA, Shetty N, Arab L: Timing of energy intake during the day is associated with the risk of obesity in adults. J Hum Nutr Diet 2014;27(suppl 2):255–262.

33 Cheng TS, Loy SL, Toh JY, Cheung YB, Chan JK, Godfrey KM, et al: Predominantly nighttime feeding and weight outcomes in infants. Am J Clin Nutr 2016;104:380–388.

34 Taveras EM, Rifas-Shiman SL, Oken E, Gunderson EP, Gillman MW: Short sleep duration in infancy and risk of childhood overweight. Arch Pediatr Adolesc Med 2008;162:305–311.

Koletzko B, Shamir R, Turck D, Phillip M (eds): Nutrition and Growth: Yearbook 2018.
World Rev Nutr Diet. Basel, Karger, 2018, vol 117, pp 129–150 (DOI: 10.1159/000484503)

Malnutrition and Catch-Up Growth during Childhood and Puberty

Michael Yackobovitch-Gavan[1] · Naama Fisch Shvalb[1] ·
Zulfiqar A. Bhutta[2,3]

[1] Jesse Z. and Sara Lea Shafer Institute of Endocrinology and Diabetes, National Center for Childhood Diabetes, Schneider Children's Medical Center of Israel, Petach Tikva, Israel; [2] Centre for Global Child Health, The Hospital for Sick Children, Toronto, ON, Canada; [3] Center of Excellence in Women and Child Health, The Aga Khan University, Karachi, Pakistan

Wasting affects an estimated 52 million children under age 5 years, and stunting, an estimated 165 million children [1]. The need for new nutritional interventions was highlighted in a recent paper on the worldwide progress towards the 2025 World Health Organization (WHO) targets for nutrition, namely, reducing and maintaining the prevalence of childhood wasting to less than 5% and reducing the number of stunted children by 40% [2]. This chapter reviews the data on malnutrition and catch-up growth published between July 1, 2016 and June 30, 2017, by topic:

1. Biomarkers of malnutrition and stunting: Three studies describing clinical and metabolic correlations that may assist clinicians in assessing the nutritional and general health status of undernourished children (Lee et al. [3], Rytter et al. [4], McGrath et al. [5]).

2. Malnutrition and the gut microbiome: Two studies reviewing the inter-relationships among malnutrition, the microbiome, and growth (Plovier and Cani [6], Velly et al. [7]).

3. Treatment of malnutrition: Six trials evaluating the effects of different interventions in the undernourished and malnourished pediatric population, 3 focused on the under-5-year age group (Dewey et al. [8], Iannotti et al. [9], Kureishy et al. [10]) and three on the over-5-year age group (Fatima et al. [11], Baum et al. [12], Ganmaa et al. [13]). Additionally, one review and one meta-analysis evaluating the impact of nutritional interventions on linear growth (Gat-Yablonski et al. [14], Roberts and Stein [15]).

4. Global aspects of treating stunting: One report on the economic implications of improving stunting (McGovern et al. [16]). One report on the investments needed to attain the WHO targets in reducing stunting (Shekar et al. [17]). One review of current thinking on the pathogenesis and risk factors for adverse developmental outcomes among young children at risk for malnutrition, setting the scene for potential interventions (Bhutta et al. [18]). One meta-analysis aimed to determine the impact that community-level sanitation access has on child stunting and health (Larsen et al. [19]).

Key articles reviewed for this chapter

The plasma proteome is associated with anthropometric status of undernourished Nepalese school-aged children

Lee SE, Stewart CP, Schulze KJ, Cole RN, Wu LS-F, Yager JD, Groopman JD, Khatry SK, Adhikari RK, Christian P, West KP Jr

J Nutr 2017;147:304–313

Correlates of thymus size and changes during treatment of children with severe acute malnutrition: a cohort study

Rytter MJ, Namusoke H, Ritz C, Michaelsen KF, Briend A, Friis H, Dorthe Jeppesen D

BMC Pediatr 2017;17:70

Biomarkers to stratify risk groups among children with malnutrition in resource-limited settings and to monitor response to intervention

McGrath CJ, Arndt MB, Walson JL

Horm Res Paediatr 2017;88:111–117

Microbial impact on host metabolism: opportunities for novel treatments of nutritional disorders?

Plovier H, Cani PD

Microbiol Spectr 2017;5:BAD-0002-2016

Mechanisms of cross-talk between the diet, the intestinal microbiome, and the under-nourished host

Velly H, Britton RA, Preidis GA

Gut Microbes 2017;8:98–112

Lipid-based nutrient supplementation in the first 1,000 days improves child growth in Bangladesh: a cluster-randomized effectiveness trial

Dewey KG, Mridha MK, Matias SL, Arnold CD, Cummins JR, Khan MS, Maalouf-Manasseh Z, Siddiqui Z, Ullah MB, Vosti SA

Am J Clin Nutr 2017;105:944–957

Eggs in early complementary feeding and child growth: a randomized controlled trial

Iannotti LL, Lutter CK, Stewart CP, Gallegos Riofrío CA, Malo C, Reinhart G, Palacios A, Karp C, Chapnick M, Cox K, Waters WF

Pediatrics 2017;140:e20163459

A mixed method study to assess the effectiveness of food-based interventions to prevent stunting among children under-five years in Districts Thatta and Sujawal, Sindh Province, Pakistan: study protocol

Kureishy S, Khan GN, Arrif S, Ashraf K, Cespedes A, Habib MA, Hussain I, Ullah A, TurabA, Ahmed I, Zaida S, Soofi SB

BMC Public Health 2017;17:24

Impact of therapeutic food compared to oral nutritional supplements on nutritional outcomes in mildly underweight healthy children in a low-medium-income society

Fatima S, Malkova D, Wright C, Gerasimidis K

Clin Nutr 2017;pii:S0261-5164(17)30097-3

The effect of egg supplementation on growth parameters in children participating in a school feeding program in rural Uganda: a pilot study

Baum JI, Miller JD, Gaines BL

Food Nutr Res 2017;61:1330097

Vitamin D supplementation and growth in urban Mongol school children: Results from two randomized clinical trials

Ganmaa D, Stuart JJ, Sumberzul N, Ninjin B, Giovannucci E, Kleinman K, Holick MF, Willett WC, Frazier LA, Rich-Edwards JW

PLoS One 2017;12:e0175237

Which dietary components modulate longitudinal growth?

Gat-Yablonski G, Yackobovitch-Gavan M, Phillip M

Curr Opin Clin Nutr Metab Care 2017;20:211–216

The impact of nutritional interventions beyond the first 2 years of life on linear growth: a systematic review and meta-analysis

Roberts JL, Stein AD

Adv Nutr 2017;8:323–336

A review of the evidence linking child stunting to economic outcomes

McGovern ME, Krishna A, Aguayo VM, Subramanian SV

Int J Epidemiol 2017;46:1171–1191

Reaching the global target to reduce stunting: an investment framework

Shekar M, Kakietek J, D'Alimonte MR, Rogers HE, Eberwein JD Akuoku JK, Pereira P, Soe-Lin S, Hecht R

Health Policy Plan 2017;32:657–668

Neurodevelopment, nutrition, and inflammation: the evolving global child health landscape

Bhutta ZA, Guerrant RL, Nelson CA

Pediatrics 2017;139(suppl 1):S12–S22

An individual-level meta-analysis assessing the impact of community-level sanitation access on child stunting, anemia, and diarrhea: evidence from DHS and MICS surveys

Larsen DA, Grisham T, Slawsky E, Narine L

PLoS Negl Trop Dis 2017;11:e0005591

The plasma proteome is associated with anthropometric status of undernourished Nepalese school-aged children

Lee SE[1], Stewart CP[2], Schulze KJ[1], Cole RN[3], Wu LS-F[1], Yager JD[4], Groopman JD[4], Khatry SK[5], Adhikari RK[6], Christian P[1], West KP Jr[1]

[1]Center for Human Nutrition, Department of International Health, Johns Hopkins Bloomberg School of Public Health, Baltimore, MD, USA; [2]Program in International and Community Nutrition, Department of Nutrition, University of California, Davis, Davis, CA, USA; [3]Mass Spectrometry and Proteomics Facility, Department of Biological Chemistry, Johns Hopkins School of Medicine, Baltimore, MD, USA; [4]Department of Environmental Health and Engineering, Johns Hopkins Bloomberg School of Public Health, Baltimore, MD, USA; [5]Nepal Nutrition Intervention Project-Sarlahi, Kathmandu, Nepal; and [6]Kathmandu Medical College, Kathmandu, Nepal

J Nutr 2017;147:304–313

Background: Our understanding of the biological pathways involved in stunting and wasting of chronically undernourished children remains insufficient. The effects of malnutrition are usually evaluated anthropometrically, but this method does not provide biological insight. Plasma proteomics may serve to highlight relevant biological pathways and single out novel protein markers of childhood growth and body composition.
Aims: To evaluate possible associations of anthropometric markers of height, musculature, and fat mass with plasma proteins in school-aged children using an untargeted proteomics approach.
Methods: A cohort of 500 Nepalese children aged 6–8 years were evaluated in this cross-sectional study. Height, weight, mid-upper arm circumference (MUAC), triceps and sub-scapular skinfolds, upper arm muscle area (AMA), and arm fat area were documented. Tandem mass spectrometry was used to measure relative plasma protein abundance. Associations between anthropometry and protein abundance were evaluated by linear mixed-effects models.
Results: Of the total 982 proteins, 1 was associated with body mass index-for-age z scores (BAZ), 10 with height-for-age z scores (HAZ), 14 with MUAC, and 17 with AMA (q < 0.05). The proteome was most robustly correlated with weight-for-age z score (WAZ; n = 33). There were strong positive associations of insulin-like growth factor (IGF)-I and its binding proteins (IGFALS and IGFBP3) with HAZ, WAZ, and AMA. Other proteins that were associated with HAZ are known to take part in nutrient transport, innate immunity, and bone mineralization. The absence of an association between proteins and measures of adiposity was noteworthy. Myosin light-chain kinase was inversely associated with BAZ, perhaps as a consequence of leakage from muscle.

Conclusions: The plasma proteomic profile was in line with recognized biomarkers of childhood growth and provided novel potential biomarkers of lean mass in children with chronic malnutrition. The suggested proteins may contribute to the assessments of growth and nutritional status of undernourished children.

Comments   Proteomics, the large-scale study of proteins, has been evolving over the past 2 decades. Although it holds promise for enhancing our understanding of biological processes, the interpretation of its findings is still challenging. Assessment of the plasma proteome specifically in undernourished children, as performed in this study, could help to focus on key proteins in lean body mass metabolism.

Besides confirming known associations between height, IGF1, and its binding proteins, this study identifies several less familiar proteins that may be of interest for future investigations: Carnosinase 1, S100A12, and Tetranectin. Carnosinase 1 is an enzyme that may be associated, based on previous studies, with muscle mass. It was found to be significantly less abundant in the plasma of stunted than non-stunted children. S100A12 has been linked to chronic intestinal inflammation in children; in this study, it was negatively associated with HAZ. Tetranectin is present in bone cartilage. It has been associated with height gain and was found to play a role in bone mineralization. These findings contribute to our investigational toolbox, although they still warrant future validation and research.

Correlates of thymus size and changes during treatment of children with severe acute malnutrition: a cohort study

Rytter MJ[1], Namusoke H[2], Ritz C[1], Michaelsen KF[1], Briend A[1,3], Friis H,[1] Dorthe Jeppesen D[4]

[1]Department of Nutrition, Exercise and Sports, University of Copenhagen, Frederiksberg C, Denmark; [2]Mwanamugimu Nutrition Unit, Mulago Hospital, Kampala, Uganda; [3]Tampere Centre for Child Health Research, University of Tampere, Tampere, Finland; [4]Department of Pediatrics, Copenhagen University Hospital Hvidovre, Copenhagen, Denmark

BMC Pediatr 2017;17:70

Background: The high rates of mortality in children with severe acute malnutrition (SAM) may be partially explained by the deleterious effects of malnutrition on the immune system. It has been suggested that thymus atrophy reflects this immunodeficiency.
Aims: To investigate associations between clinical and nutritional measures and thymus size in children with SAM and to describe factors affecting the increase in thymus size during nutritional intervention.
Methods: The cohort of this observational study, performed in Uganda, comprised of children with SAM, aged 6–59 months, who were hospitalized for nutritional treatment. The thymus area was measured by ultrasound on admission, at discharge, and after 8 weeks of nutritional intervention with ready-to-use therapeutic food (RUTF; F-75 or F-100 formulas). Findings were compared with healthy, adequately nourished children. Anthropometric and biochemical markers of nutritional status were measured and correlated with thymus size and growth.
Results: Eighty-five malnourished children of median age 16.5 months were included in the study. The median thymus area was significantly smaller in the malnourished than the healthy children ($p < 0.001$); in 27% of the malnourished children, the thymus was undetectable on ultrasound at admission. There was a significant correlation of thymus area with WAZ and mid-upper-arm-

circumference as well as with levels of serum hemoglobin and plasma phosphate. Thymus area was negatively associated with illness severity (as assessed by caretakers) and elevated inflammatory markers. After 8 weeks of nutritional rehabilitation, the thymus area increased dramatically ($p < 0.001$), in accordance with an increase in mid-upper-arm-circumference. There was a lesser increase in thymus area in children in whom the F-75 formula was partially replaced with rice porridge during their hospital stay.

Conclusions: Thymus atrophy is a marker of malnutrition and inflammation in children with SAM, and is reversible under optimal nutritional rehabilitation. The correlation between plasma phosphate levels and thymus size should be further explored to improve our understanding of their possible mutual effects.

Comments   This study was prompted by earlier reports of an association between undernutrition and reversible thymus atrophy [20, 21]. The authors sought to identify specific clinical and biochemical correlates of thymus area and predictors of thymus area growth during nutritional rehabilitation. The study confirms the reduction in thymus size in nutritional deprivation and inflammation and adds a novel finding of a positive correlation of thymus size with hemoglobin and phosphate levels. The correlation with phosphate levels is supported by the finding that the children who received the nutritionally inferior rice porridge had both reduced thymus growth and a slower increase in plasma phosphate, and raises a question regarding the role of phosphate in thymus growth and function. In a parallel study on this cohort, the authors found that the children fed with the poorer diet, who had a lower phosphate level on day 2, also had a higher rate of mortality [22]. Further research is needed to determine if thymus atrophy is involved in the pathogenesis of malnutrition and/or inflammation or if it is only a marker of these conditions, and to identify the mechanism whereby nutritional rehabilitation leads to an increase in thymus size.

Biomarkers to stratify risk groups among children with malnutrition in resource-limited settings and to monitor response to intervention

McGrath CJ[1], Arndt MB[2], Walson JL[3]

[1]Department of Obstetrics and Gynecology, University of Texas Medical Branch, Galveston, TX, USA; [2]PATH, Seattle, WA, USA; [3]Departments of Global Health, Pediatrics, Medicine, and Epidemiology, University of Washington, Seattle, WA, USA; The Childhood Acute Illness and Nutrition Network (CHAIN), Nairobi, Kenya

Horm Res Paediatr 2017;88:111–117

Although substantial efforts are being directed at lowering rates of childhood undernutrition, interventions so far have not been as effective as expected and gaps remain in our understanding of the mechanisms underlying stunting. Tools are needed to identify the children who are more likely to respond to nutritional rehabilitation in addition to markers of response to treatment.

Environmental enteral dysfunction (EED) is a subclinical intestinal disorder that affects many children in low-income countries. EED may worsen malnutrition and contribute to the risk of morbidity and mortality in affected children. Alongside EED, changes and insults to the gut flora in the early years of life may lead to impaired growth owing to their adverse effects on nutrient absorption, metabolism, local inflammatory responses, and hormonal regulation.

This review describes the current knowledge on the interplay between EED, the gut microbiome, and impaired linear growth in malnourished children. It highlights novel biomarkers that may help distinguish children at higher risk of malnutrition and to measure the response to nutritional interventions.

Comments This review provides a comprehensive overview of the many biomarkers of growth failure in malnourished children investigated to date. These include urinary, stool, and plasma markers of the different stages of EED (increased intestinal permeability, epithelial damage and repair, gut inflammation, and microbial translocation) as well as markers of microbiome dysfunction, systemic inflammation, and resistance to growth hormone. Because stunting is the result of a series of complex processes, none of these individual markers has the power to predict clinical outcome, and a composite score of several markers might serve as a more efficient tool.

Microbial impact on host metabolism: opportunities for novel treatments of nutritional disorders?

Plovier H[1, 2], Cani PD[1, 2]

[1]WELBIO – Walloon Excellence in Life Sciences and Biotechnology and [2]Metabolism and Nutrition Research Group, Louvain Drug Research Institute, Université Catholique de Louvain, Brussels, Belgium

Microbiol Spectr 2017;5:BAD-0002-2016

Malnutrition has an impact not only on the human organs but also on the normal development of the human gut microbiota. Studies comparing the relative abundance of different gut bacteria show substantial differences in the microbiome between healthy and undernourished children.
Normally, the gut microbiome evolves during the first 3 years of life before reaching the composition observed in adults. Nutritional deficiencies have been shown to alter the relative abundance of different bacterial species within the microbiome, delaying or disrupting this process. The immature microbiota may adversely affect intestinal absorption and take part in the pathogenesis of stunting and wasting seen in malnourished children. This review discusses the involvement of the gut microbiome both in states of undernutrition and in obesity and metabolic syndrome and presents possible therapeutic uses of gut microbes for these nutritional disorders.

Mechanisms of cross-talk between the diet, the intestinal microbiome, and the under-nourished host

Velly H[1], Britton RA[1], Preidis GA[2]

[1]Center for Metagenomics and Microbiome Research, Department of Molecular Virology and Microbiology, Baylor College of Medicine, Houston, TX, USA; [2]Section of Gastroenterology, Hepatology, and Nutrition, Department of Pediatrics, Baylor College of Medicine and Texas Children's Hospital, Houston, TX, USA

Gut Microbes 2017;8:98–112

Imbalances in the gut microbiome are emerging as an important contributor to the deleterious effects of malnutrition on child growth. Observational studies show that specific changes occur in the microbial community in undernourished children, with a decreased variance and richness of taxa and a different relative abundance of various microbial species compared to healthy children. Besides malnutrition, these disruptions also result in decreased resistance to entero-pathogenic bacteria and directly interfere with weight gain and longitudinal growth. This review describes recent studies of alterations in the gut microbiome in malnourished children; outlines the dietary, environmental, and host factors that influence the microbiome; explains the outcomes of dysbiosis on normal physiology, and discusses the various current treatment options, future challenges, and opportunities in this field.

Comments   These 2 reviews taken together provide a comprehensive synopsis of the known associations among the gut microbes, undernutrition, and growth. Both discuss the effects of diet on normal microbiome development, including the contribution of human milk oligosaccharides on priming of the microbiome, and present interventional trials targeted at the microbiome which have had limited success so far. Future therapeutic options based on animal models are suggested. The review of Plovier and Cani [6] proposes an interesting connection between 2 seemingly opposite conditions: undernutrition and obesity/ metabolic syndrome. Both are characterized by imbalances in the gut microbiome, leading to increased inflammatory potential, a reduced diversity of gut microbiota, and decreased ecological fitness (impaired resistance to colonization). The review by Velly et al. [7] offers a more in-depth description of the mechanisms whereby intestinal dysbiosis develops and the ways in which it may participate in the pathogenesis of stunting in the undernourished host. The shortcomings of current treatment options are discussed along with potential means of overcoming them.

Lipid-based nutrient supplementation in the first 1,000 days improves child growth in Bangladesh: a cluster-randomized effectiveness trial

Dewey KG[1], Mridha MK[1, 4], Matias SL[1], Arnold CD[1], Cummins JR[3], Khan MS[5], Maalouf-Manasseh Z[6], Siddiqui Z[4], Ullah MB[1], Vosti SA[2]

Departments of [1]Nutrition and [2]Agricultural and Resource Economics, University of California at Davis, Davis, CA, USA; [3]Department of Economics, University of California, Riverside, CA, USA; [4]Nutrition and Clinical Science Division and [5]Initiative of Noncommunicable Disease, Health Systems and Population Studies Division, icddr,b, Dhaka, Bangladesh; and [6]Food and Nutrition Technical Assistance III Project (FANTA)/FHI 360, Washington, DC, USA

Am J Clin Nutr 2017;105:944–957

Background: Stunting during the first 1,000 days of life is very common in developing countries. In Bangladesh, 36% of all children under age 5 years show stunted growth [23]. The need for new nutritional interventions to reduce this prevalence was highlighted in a recent paper on the 2025 WHO targets for nutrition [2].

Aims: To assess the effect of different home fortification approaches on linear growth and head size from birth to 24 months.

Methods: A researcher-blind, longitudinal, cluster-randomized effectiveness trial was conducted. The population included 4,011 women at ≤20 weeks of gestation within 64 clusters. The interventions (4 arms) were offered to mothers during pregnancy and the first 6 months postpartum and/ or to their children, from age 6 to 24 months, as follows:

1. Women and children both received lipid-based nutrient supplements (LNS; 118 kcal, about 10 g fat, 2.6 g protein, multi-vitamins and minerals – different doses in mothers vs. children; LNS-LNS group).

2. Women received iron and folic acid (IFA, 1 tablet of 60 mg Fe and 400 mg folic acid) and children received LNS (IFA-LNS group).

3. Women received IFA and children received micronutrient powder (MNP; containing 15 micronutrients; IFA-MNP group).

4. Women received IFA and children received no supplements (IFA-Control group).

Results: A total of 3,379 participants completed the study. At age 24 months, mean length-for-age z score (LAZ) was significantly higher (+0.13) in children exposed to both prenatal and postnatal LNS (LNS-LNS) than in children given MNP (IFA-MNP), with no differences between the LNS-LNS and IFA-LNS groups (–1.72 and –1.73, respectively). Although children exposed only to postnatal LNS had a slightly lower mean LAZ at birth (–0.09) than children exposed to LNS both pre- and postnatally, by 24 months, LAZ was similar in the 2 groups. At 18 months, the prevalence of stunting (LAZ <–2) was lower in the LNS-LNS group than in the IFA-MNP group (OR 0.70; 95% CI 0.53–0.92), but the difference diminished by 24 months (OR 0.81; 95% CI 0.63–1.04). The mean head-circumference-for-age z score at 24 months was significantly higher (+0.14) in the LNS-LNS than the IFA-control group.

Conclusions: The results suggest that there are modest improvements in linear growth status and head size in undernourished children given LNS during the first 2 years of life, but not in undernourished children given MNP for the same period.

Comments This large interventional cluster-randomized controlled study by Dewey et al. [8] assessed the effect of different home fortification approaches on growth from birth to 2 years of life in undernourished newborns from Bangladesh. There were modest improvements in linear growth status and head size at 2 years in the children fed LNS (LNS-containing 118 kcal, about 10 g fat, 2.6 g protein, multi-vitamins and minerals) but not in children fed MNP (MNP-containing 15 micronutrients). Giving mothers LNS prenatally yielded no advantage in growth outcomes of their offspring at 2 years. These findings suggest that differences in the nutrient content between LNS and MNP may account for the differences in length-for-age between the LNS-LNS and IFA-MNP groups. However, as pointed out also by the authors, the micronutrient content of the LNS and MNP supplements differed as well, making it impossible to isolate the specific nutrients that were most critical to the improved growth in the LNS-exposed children. LNS provided energy, macronutrients, and several vitamins and minerals (calcium, potassium, phosphorus, magnesium, pantothenic acid, vitamin K) that were not included in MNP. In addition, the LNS supplement contained more zinc (8 compared with 4.1 mg), selenium (20 compared with 17 mg), and vitamin E (6 compared with 5 mg). The most likely candidates contributing to the postnatal linear growth response are energy, macronutrients, and macrominerals (calcium, potassium, phosphorus, magnesium). The dietary fat in the LNS supplements may have played a key role as well, given the importance of polyunsaturated fatty acids for brain development, immune function, and growth [24–26].

The impact of fortified supplements such as LNS containing mixtures of macronutrients and micronutrients should continue to be evaluated in the context of broader strategies to reduce stunting.

Eggs in early complementary feeding and child growth: a randomized controlled trial

Iannotti LL[1], Lutter CK[2], Stewart CP[3], Gallegos Riofrío CA[4], Malo C[4], Reinhart G[5], Palacios A[5], Karp C[4], Chapnick M[1], Cox K[1], Waters WF[4]

[1]Brown School, Institute for Public Health, Washington University in St Louis, St Louis, MO, USA; [2]School of Public Health, University of Maryland, College Park, MD, USA; [3]Department of Nutrition, University of California, Davis, Davis, CA, USA; [4]Institute for Research in Health and Nutrition, Universidad San Francisco de Quito, Quito, Pichincha, Ecuador; [5]The Mathile Institute for the Advancement of Human Nutrition, Dayton, OH, USA

Pediatrics 2017;140(1):e20163459

This manuscript is also discussed in Chapter 9, pages 165–175.

Background: Most interventions aimed at reducing stunting have used micronutrient-fortified foods or supplements composed of combinations of macronutrients and micronutrients. Evidence for the effectiveness of locally available nutritious foods is limited. Eggs are an affordable and feasible source of nutrients such as high-quality protein, vitamin B12, zinc and iron, important for growth and development.
Aims: The aim of the study was to evaluate the growth-related effect of feeding children with one egg per day for 6 months, starting at age 6–9 months.
Methods: A randomized controlled trial was conducted in Ecuador over a 6-month period. Children aged 6–9 months were randomly assigned to intervention ($n = 83$) and nonintervention (control; $n = 80$) groups. The intervention consisted of 1 medium-sized egg (~50 g) per day for 6 months; the eggs were supplied to the treatment group on a weekly basis. Children in the control group were visited every week and monitored for morbidities. The primary outcomes were changes in anthropometric measures of child growth between baseline and at the end of the intervention. Secondary end points were dietary intake, allergy symptoms, and morbidity symptoms.
Results: The baseline prevalence of stunting was 38%, and the mean length-for-age z score (LAZ) was -1.90 ± 1.01. At baseline, the intervention group had a higher prevalence of stunting and underweight than the control group. At the end of 6 months, the intervention group had a higher LAZ than the control group by 0.63 (95% CI 0.38–0.88) and a higher WAZ by 0.61 (95% CI 0.45–0.77). In addition, the intervention resulted in significant reductions of 47% in the prevalence of stunting (prevalence ratio [PR]) 0.53; 95% CI 0.37–0.77) and of 74% in the prevalence of underweight (PR 0.26; 95% CI 0.10–0.70). Besides their higher dietary intake of eggs (PR 1.57; 95% CI 1.28–1.92), the intervention group had a better dietary composition than controls, including reduced intake of sugar-sweetened foods (PR 0.71; 95% CI 0.51–0.97). No allergic reactions to the eggs were reported during the study.
Conclusions: An affordable and feasible food-based intervention of one egg per day for 6 months beginning at age 6–9 months had a significant positive effect on linear growth and weight gain in a resource-poor pediatric population. These results indicate that eggs have the potential to contribute to global targets to reduce stunting.

Comments Most of the earlier studies on the effect of nutritional intervention on catch-up growth in young children from resource-poor populations used supplements containing mixtures of micronutrients or combinations of both macro- and micronutrients. Eggs are an accessible complete food, rich in growth-promoting nutrients, including high-quality protein, with high concentrations of choline and other micronutrients such as vitamin B12, zinc, and iron. This randomized controlled trial in an Andean pediatric population demonstrated that 6 months of complementary feeding with 1 egg per day starting as early as age 6–9 months, significantly improved the linear growth (increase in LAZ by 0.63 and in WAZ by 0.61) and reduced stunting. Effect sizes for the anthropometric outcomes were similar to those reported for protein supplements in the 2017 meta-analysis by Roberts and Stein (presented later in this chapter; mean effect size, 0.68), and stronger than reported for interventions including multiple micronutrients (mean effect size, 0.26) or a single micronutrient (mean effect size: zinc –0.15, vitamin A –0.05). These results should be validated in larger studies in different pediatric populations.

A mixed methods study to assess the effectiveness of food-based interventions to prevent stunting among children under-five years in Districts Thatta and Sujawal, Sindh Province, Pakistan: study protocol

Kureishy S[1], Khan GN[1], Arrif S[1], Ashraf K[2], Cespedes A[2], Habib MA[1], Hussain I[1], Ullah A[1], Turab A[1], Ahmed I[1], Zaida S[3], Soofi SB[1]

[1]Department of Paediatrics and Child Health, Aga Khan University, Karachi, Pakistan; [2]World Food Programme, Islamabad, Pakistan; [3]Department of Community Health Sciences, Aga Khan University, Karachi, Pakistan

BMC Public Health 2017;17:24

Background: The high prevalence of maternal and child malnutrition in low- and middle-income developing countries poses a major challenge. Child malnutrition is attributed to poverty, absence of appropriate child-care practices, poor diet quality, and recurring infections during the first 2 years of life. It has both short- and long-term adverse effects on outcomes, including stunting and wasting, short adult stature, intellectual disability, reduced educational achievements, and lower earnings [27, 28]. It is therefore important to identify effective preventive approaches.

Aims: We present a study proposal with the primary aim of evaluating the effectiveness of food-based interventions to reduce stunting in children aged 6–59 months at risk of malnutrition residing in low- and middle-income countries. The secondary aim is to assess the effect of food-based interventions on micronutrient deficiencies, wasting, anemia, and rates of low birth weight.

Methods: A mixed-methods study design will be used in 3 different settings: (1) a cross-sectional survey of 7,360 study participants; (2) a community-based cluster randomized controlled trial with 5,000 participants; (3) a process evaluation of the acceptability, feasibility, and potential barriers of project implementation through focus group discussions, key informant interviews, and household surveys.

The study participants will include pregnant women and lactating mothers and children less than 5 years old from the Thatta and Sujawal Districts of Sindh Province, Pakistan. The randomized control trial will consist of 3 arms, as follows: (1) children aged 6–23 months given locally produced LNS; (2) children aged 24–59 months given MNP; (3) pregnant and lactating mothers given wheat soya blend. All food-based supplements will be delivered by healthcare workers using a blanket approach. The control group will receive routine public and private health services available within the area. Study participants will be followed monthly for compliance with the supplements, dietary diversity, pregnancy outcomes, and maternal and child morbidity and mortality. Anthropometric parameters and hemoglobin levels will be measured at baseline, quarterly, and at the end of follow-up.

Comments Various food-based interventions for maternal and child malnutrition have been evaluated to date in developing countries, including LNS, fortified blended foods, and

MNP. All showed positive effects on child health and growth [29]. However, studies were usually conducted in controlled environments, and the results could not be generalized to programs operating under field conditions.

In the present large community-based study, the authors aim to evaluate the effectiveness of food-based interventions on reducing stunting among children less than 5 years old from low- and middle-income countries who are at risk of malnutrition. The major strengths of this study are the large cohort, the mixed-methods design including a cross-sectional survey, a community-based cluster-randomized controlled trial, and a process evaluation, and the joint interventions in the mothers and children. The results may provide sufficient evidence for the development of policies and programs designed to improve growth outcomes in the pediatric population in poor resource settings.

Impact of therapeutic food compared to oral nutritional supplements on nutritional outcomes in mildly underweight healthy children in a low-medium-income society

Fatima S[1,2], Malkova D[1], Wright C[1], Gerasimidis K[1]

[1]School of Medicine, Dentistry and Nursing, College of Medical, Veterinary and Life Sciences, University of Glasgow, UK; [2]Khyber Medical University, Peshawar, Pakistan

Clin Nutr 2017;pii:S0261-5164(17)30097-3

Background: RUTF is an energy-dense paste that can be stored at room temperature for several months and eaten without the addition of water or milk, thereby reducing the risk of contamination. In children 5 years old or less from low- and middle-income countries, where malnutrition is highly prevalent, RUTF is frequently used for the treatment of severe acute malnutrition. Young children living in more affluent countries are usually given liquid oral nutritional supplements (ONS) to treat disease-associated malnutrition and poor appetite. The effectiveness of these strategies has not been studied in older children, or for long-term effect in moderate malnutrition.

Aims: This study compared the effects of RUTF and ONS on growth parameters in mildly underweight primary school children living in a low-/middle-income country.

Methods: Sixty-eight mildly underweight (weight z score, –2 to –1) Pakistani children aged 5–10 years (93% girls) were recruited and randomized to 4 weeks' intervention with either RUTF or ONS (500 kcal/day), in addition to their regular diet. Height, weight, and subscapular and triceps skinfold thickness were measured at baseline, at the end of the intervention (4 weeks), and again 15 months later. The primary outcome measure was the difference in the change in weight z score between the 2 groups after 4 weeks of supplementation. Secondary outcomes were differences in the changes in height z score, BMI z score, and skinfold z score.

Results: After 4 weeks of intervention, the nutritional status improved in both groups. There were no significant between-group differences in any of the primary and secondary outcome measures. The average weight gain in both groups was 0.6 kg, which was lower than anticipated (2 kg). At 15 months after supplementation, there was a tendency for weight z scores and height z scores to return to baseline.

Conclusions: Intervention with RUTF and ONS produced a similar gain in weight and height in children aged 5–10 years at risk of malnutrition. The effect of both supplements was lower than expected and tended not to persist after supplementation was stopped.

Comments This is an important attempt to find the best nutritional intervention for catch-up growth in undernourished children. The authors compared the effects of 4 weeks of treatment with RUTF or ONS on growth parameters in mildly underweight primary school children and found that both interventions had a similar small positive effect on weight and height gain. The main strength of this study was the high compliance and low drop-out rate relative to other similar studies. This was achieved by conducting the intervention in a primary school during the school year, having the supplements delivered to the children at school every morning, and asking the children to consume the supplements in addition to their regular diet.

However, this study has several limitations. Most important, owing to the absence of an untreated control (preferably placebo-treated) group, it was impossible to determine if the gains in weight and height were a true effect of treatment or attributable to other factors such as seasonal variation. Furthermore, the duration of the intervention (4 weeks) was probably too short to produce a significant effect on growth or to yield significant between-group differences. The children's regular dietary intake was not assessed at baseline or during the intervention, so the actual extent of the dietary compensation could not be estimated. This could explain the relatively small effect on weight gain. Other limitations include the small number of participants, their narrow age range, and the predominance of girls (93%), which preclude extrapolation of the findings to older age groups or to boys.

More studies are needed to establish the best composition and the best way of delivery of supplements targeted to induce catch-up growth in undernourished children.

The effect of egg supplementation on growth parameters in children participating in a school feeding program in rural Uganda: a pilot study

Baum JI[1], Miller JD[2], Gaines BL[1]

[1]Department of Food Science, University of Arkansas, Fayetteville, AR, USA; [2]Department of Agricultural Education, Communications and Technology, University of Arkansas, Fayetteville, AR, USA

Food Nutr Res 2017;61:1330097

Background: School feeding programs have gained popularity in developing countries. Eggs are an inexpensive source of micronutrients and high-quality protein. Therefore, the objective of this study was to gain preliminary data regarding the impact of egg supplementation on growth in primary school students participating in a school feeding program in rural Uganda.

Methods: Children (ages 6–9; $n = 241$) were recruited from 3 different schools located in the Kitgum District of Uganda. All participants in the same school received the same dietary intervention: control (no eggs [0 eggs]; $n = 56$), one egg 5 days per week (1 egg; $n = 89$), or 2 eggs 5 days per week (2 eggs; $n = 96$). Height, weight, triceps skinfold thickness, and MUAC were measured monthly over 6 months.

Results: Following 6 months of egg supplementation, participants receiving 2 eggs had a greater increase in height and weight compared to the 0 eggs and 1 egg groups ($p < 0.05$). In addition, participants receiving 1 egg and 2 eggs had a significantly higher ($p < 0.05$) increase in MUAC at 6 months compared to 0 eggs.

Conclusion: These results suggest that supplementation with eggs can improve parameters of growth in school-aged children participating in school feeding programs in rural Uganda.

Comments This is an important corroborative study of the value of school age nutrition on growth parameters in African children, supporting the improved growth seen in young infants in Ecuador with egg-based complementary feeding by Iannotti et al. [9], reviewed earlier in this chapter. The findings that eggs can provide an important source of quality protein in older children, also associated with improved linear growth, are notable in that they support the continuation of nutrition programs beyond the preschool period in vulnerable populations. The dose-related effects are also supportive of measures to ensure optimal protein intake in such children and similar findings with improved weight gain and hemoglobin have been reported from older school children in China [30].

Vitamin D supplementation and growth in urban Mongol school children: Results from two randomized clinical trials

Ganmaa D[1–3], Stuart JJ[4, 5], Sumberzul N[3], Ninjin B[3], Giovannucci E[1, 2, 4], Kleinman K[6], Holick MF[7], Willett WC[1, 2, 4], Frazier LA[1, 4, 8], Rich-Edwards JW[1, 4, 5]

[1]Channing Laboratory, Brigham and Women's Hospital, Harvard Medical School, Boston, MA, USA; [2]Department of Nutrition, Harvard T.H. Chan School of Public Health, Boston, MA, USA; [3]Health Sciences University of Mongolia, Ulaanbaatar, Mongolia; [4]Department of Epidemiology, Harvard T.H. Chan School of Public Health, Boston, MA, USA; [5]Connors Center for Women's Health and Gender Biology, Brigham and Women's Hospital, Boston, MA, United States of America. [6]Population Medicine, Harvard Pilgrim Health Care Institute and Harvard Medical School, Boston, MA, USA; [7]Endocrine, Diabetes and Nutrition Section, Department of Medicine, Boston University Medical Center, Boston, MA, USA; [8]Department of Pediatric Oncology, Dana Farber Cancer Institute, Boston, MA, USA

PLoS One 2017;12:e0175237

Background: Symptomatic vitamin D deficiency is associated with slowed growth in children. It is unknown whether vitamin D repletion in children with asymptomatic serum vitamin D deficiency can restore normal growth.

Objective: We tested the impact of vitamin D-supplementation on serum concentrations of 25-hydroxyvitamin D and short-term growth in Mongol children, with very low serum vitamin D levels in winter.

Design: We conducted 2 randomized, double-blind, placebo-controlled trials in urban school age children without clinical signs of rickets. The Supplementation Study was a 6-month intervention with an 800 IU vitamin D3 supplement daily, compared with placebo, in 113 children aged 12–15 years. A second study, the Fortification Study, was a 7-week intervention with 710 mL of whole milk fortified with 300 IU vitamin D3 daily, compared with unfortified milk, in 235 children aged 9–11 years.

Results: At winter baseline, children had low vitamin D levels, with a mean (±SD) serum 25-hydroxyvitamin D concentration of 7.3 (±3.9) ng/mL in the supplementation study and 7.5 (±3.8) ng/mL in the fortification study. The serum levels increased in both vitamin D groups – by 19.8 (±5.1) ng/mL in the Supplementation Study, and 19.7 (±6.1) ng/mL in the fortification study. Multivariable analysis showed a 0.9 (±0.3 SE) cm increase in height in the vitamin-D treated children, compared to placebo-treated children, in the 6-month supplementation study ($p = 0.003$). Although the children in the 7-week fortification study intervention arm grew 0.2 (±0.1) cm more, on average, than placebo children, this difference was not statistically significant ($p = 0.2$).

Yackobovitch-Gavan · Fisch Shvalb · Bhutta

There were no significant effects of vitamin D supplements on differences in changes in weight or body mass index in either trial. For the fortification study, girls gained more weight than boys while taking vitamin D3 (*p* value for interaction = 0.03), but sex was not an effect modifier of the relationship between vitamin D3 and change in either height or BMI in either trial.

Conclusions: Correcting vitamin D deficiency in children with very low serum vitamin D levels using 800 IU of vitamin D3 daily for 6 months increased growth, at least in the short-term, whereas, in a shorter trial of 300 IU of D fortified milk daily for 7 weeks it did not.

Comments   This study in a population with endemic vitamin D deficiency demonstrates how studies ought to have the appropriate power to evaluate the impact of appropriate doses of vitamin D by high-risk groups and dose-dependent effects, even among older school children. The role of vitamin D in maternal health and child growth and development merits definitive large-scale evaluations, including placebo-controlled trials, with appropriate follow-up information and end points. Designing such studies in populations with endemic deficiencies poses significant ethical challenges and might require the use of quasi-experimental designs or pragmatic incremental adaptive designs. Other studies have failed to find an association between vitamin D status in infancy and growth and morbidity in childhood [31], supported by other studies in Asia [32], although at variance with findings from the ALSPAC cohort [33] which found associations with maternal vitamin D status in pregnancy and neurodevelopmental outcomes in pre-school children. Other studies in India have documented associations between vitamin D status in young children and growth and morbidity [34], underscoring the need for larger, well-designed multi-country evaluation of the role of maternal and infant vitamin D status in affecting childhood morbidity, growth, and neurodevelopment.

Which dietary components modulate longitudinal growth?

Gat-Yablonski G[1–3], Yackobovitch-Gavan M[1], Phillip M[1–3]

[1]National Center for Childhood Diabetes, Schneider Children's Medical Center of Israel, The Jesse Z and Sara Lea Shafer Institute for Endocrinology and Diabetes, Petach Tikva, Israel; [2]Sackler Faculty of Medicine, Tel Aviv University, Tel Aviv, Israel; [3]Felsenstein Medical Research Center, Petach Tikva, Israel

Curr Opin Clin Nutr Metab Care 2017;20:211–216

This review, recently published by our group, aimed to summarize the most recent knowledge on the role of nutrition in the process of linear growth. Included were peer-reviewed papers mostly published from 2014 onward that explored the effects of macronutrients (specifically, protein and fat), micronutrients (specifically, zinc, iron and iodine), and different nutritional combinations on catch-up growth in undernourished children and food-restricted animal models. Some interesting recent studies regarding the effect of different sources of proteins and specific amino acids were presented.

Comments   The well-recognized presence of a link between nutrition and linear growth in children is based on the intuitive wisdom of countless generations. However, only recently has substantial progress been made in clarifying the mechanisms underlying this association and the role of nutrition in catch-up growth.

Various nutritional components serve as essential building blocks for growing tissues. They participate in growth regulation by acting as regulatory agents in the epiphyseal growth plate and by influencing the gut microbiome. Studies have shown that nutritional supplementation with a mixture of macronutrients and micronutrients is more beneficial than supplementation with a single nutrient. However, much work is still required to establish the nutritional composition that produces the best outcomes for catch-up growth without long-term metabolic complications.

The impact of nutritional interventions beyond the first 2 years of life on linear growth: a systematic review and meta-analysis

Roberts JL[1], Stein AD[1, 2]

[1]Nutrition and Health Sciences, Laney Graduate School and [2]Hubert Department of Global Health, Rollins School of Public Health, Emory University, Atlanta, GA, USA

Adv Nutr 2017;8:323–336

Background: There is a large body of evidence emphasizing the importance of nutritional interventions early in life for the prevention and treatment of malnutrition and stunting. However, several recent publications indicate that catch-up growth also occurs after infancy, and suggest that it may be possible to promote catch-up growth even beyond this early window [35, 36].

Aims: The aim of this systematic review was to evaluate the effectiveness of different nutrition-based interventions on linear growth in children ≥2 years of age.

Methods: A systematic search of MEDLINE and EMBASE (1947–2016) was performed using the keywords "nutrition and height and growth". The primary response variable was a change in height (in centimeters) or height z score.

Results: A total of 69 studies met the inclusion criteria. The meta-analyses showed that protein supplementation had the strongest significant positive effects on linear growth (mean effect size 0.68; 95% CI 0.30–1.05), followed by multiple micronutrients (mean effect size, 0.26; 95% CI 0.13–0.39). In addition, single-micronutrient intervention with zinc (mean effect size, 0.15; 95% CI 0.06–0.24) and vitamin A (mean effect size, 0.05; 95% CI 0.01–0.09) had significant small positive effects on linear growth. Other nutritional interventions, including iron, calcium, and iodine, and food-based interventions had no significant effect on growth. Baseline height-SD score was a significant inverse predictor of the effect size. Baseline age, study duration, and dose were not related to effect size for any nutrient examined.

Conclusions: Adequate nutritional intervention, specifically with protein, multiple micronutrients, zinc, and vitamin A, has the potential to improve linear growth after age 2 years, especially in children with growth failure.

Comments This systematic review by Roberts and Stein is important because it shows that the window of opportunity to address stunting does not close at 2 years of age, and adequate nutritional intervention, specifically protein, multiple micronutrients, zinc and vitamin A, has the potential to induce catch-up growth, especially in undernourished children with stunting.

This review highlights several limitations of the existing literature. First, approximately half of the included trials were of medium to low quality, as assessed by Jadad scoring (no randomization, no double-blind design, and/or no description of withdrawals and dropouts). Second, the duration of most of the trials was less than 12 months, which may not be long enough to observe a significant effect on linear growth. Third, in each of the meta-analyses, there was a large heterogeneity among the included studies in terms of supplement composition and dose, duration of the intervention, and demographic and clinical characteristics of the participants. This made it difficult to determine the best intervention (composition and dose), the population most likely to benefit (baseline age, anthropometric and other clinical characteristics), and the expected effect size.

Future high quality and long-term (>12 months) interventional studies that include different pediatric populations from both developing and developed countries are needed to improve our understanding of the effect of different dietary components on linear growth.

A review of the evidence linking child stunting to economic outcomes

McGovern ME[1, 2], Krishna A[3, 4], Aguayo VM[5], Subramanian SV[3, 4]

[1]CHaRMS: Centre for Health Research at the Management School, and [2]UKCRC Centre of Excellence for Public Health, Queen's University, Belfast, Northern Ireland; [3]Harvard Center for Population and Development Studies and [4]Department of Social and Behavioral Sciences, Harvard T.H. Chan School of Public Health, Boston, MA, USA; [5]United Nations Children's Fund (UNICEF), Nutrition Section, Programme Division, New York, NY, USA

Int J Epidemiol 2017;46:1171–1191

Background: Childhood undernutrition and subsequent stunting may have long-term economic nationwide implications which may, in turn, influence the decisions of policy-makers regarding the allocation of resources towards prevention.

Aims: This study aims to provide accurate information on the long-term cost-effectiveness of intervention programs aimed at reducing childhood undernutrition on a personal and a national level.

Methods: A literature search was conducted for studies focused on childhood stunting and its physical or economic outcomes in adulthood. The strength of the evidence tying the prevalence of stunting to economic growth was evaluated, and the implications of the findings for countries with a high rate of childhood undernutrition were summarized.

Results: Two randomized interventional trials with long-term follow-up showed a significant 25 and 46% increase in wages for adults who had been in the intervention arms. Quasi-experimental studies evaluating the influence of adult height on wages found a median increase of 4% per centimeter for men and 6% for women. Cost-benefit analyses of nutritional interventions demonstrated a median return of 17.9:1 per child. However, an increase in gross domestic product was not unequivocally associated with a reduction in childhood stunting.

Conclusions: Countries afflicted by large-scale childhood stunting should regard policies and programs directed at treating child undernutrition as a cost-beneficial allocation of resources with a high return on the investment. Aiming at general economic growth is probably not effective on its own in reducing the prevalence of stunting unless relevant issues that contribute to childhood malnutrition are specifically addressed.

Reaching the global target to reduce stunting: an investment framework

Shekar M[1], Kakietek J[1], D'Alimonte MR[2], Rogers HE[2], Eberwein JD[1] Akuoku JK[1], Pereira P[1], Soe-Lin S[2], Hecht R[2]

[1]Health, Nutrition and Population Global Practice, World Bank, Washington, DC, USA; [2]Results for Development, Washington, DC, USA

Health Policy Plan 2017;32:657–668

Background: Stunting in the first years of life is associated with poorer cognitive development, lower intelligence scores, and a reduction of 5–53% in adult wages. The effect of these personal consequences on economic growth has prompted large-scale investments in nutritional interventions, which have been shown to be cost-effective. In 2015, the World Health Assembly set a series of 10-year global nutrition targets, including a reduction of 40% in the number of children less than 5 years old with stunting.

Aims: To assess the required increase in funding of stunting prevention needed to reach global nutrition targets, and to suggest financing scenarios that may help achieve this goal.

Methods: The analysis focused on interventions with a strong proof of success in reducing stunting. The required annual increase in costs for a sample of 37 countries carrying the highest rates of stunting was estimated, and the effect of the budget scale-up on stunting prevalence was evaluated using the Lives Saved Tool model. Estimates of current spending on key interventions were derived from data on government, donors, and household expenditures. Finally, 2 financing scenarios were modeled: "business as usual," an extension of current financing, and "global solidarity," a plan for coordinated additional funding from all sources.

Results: The financial requirement for reaching the 2025 target by intervention scale-up is USD 49.5 billion. The annual average increase in funding required ranges from USD 2.6 billion to USD 7.4 billion. The "business as usual" scenario was not sufficient, and the target was not met.

Conclusions: Achieving the global target of a reduction in stunting is possible, but coordinated global investment and careful planning are required.

Comments These 2 studies deal with the economic aspects of treating malnutrition. McGovern et al. [16] conducted a comprehensive assessment of the financial benefit of reducing the rate of stunting. There are very few long-term follow-up studies on randomized nutritional interventions in childhood that provide high-quality evidence of the productivity of the affected children as adults. Non-interventional prospective studies and cross-sectional studies should be interpreted more cautiously for obvious methodological reasons. McGovern et al. [16] reevaluated the data derived from previous studies to assess the impact of stunting on economic productivity and improve our understanding of the economic implications of malnutrition. They concluded that a reduction in the prevalence of stunting is likely to yield substantial returns to society. This valuable information is encouraging to policy planners in low-income countries. Another important conclusion of this study is that merely improving the per capita gross domestic product of a country is unlikely to affect the rate of stunting, and only targeted investments in nutrition programs, gender equality issues, and sanitation will result in true improvement. This study sends a practical, well-based message to health policy planners across the world on the importance and significance of treating childhood malnutrition.

The second study, by Shekar et al. [17], sought to provide a practical framework for reaching the WHO global nutrition target of a 40% reduction in stunting by 2025, in terms of both cost and informed selection of effective interventions. For instance, the authors recommend investing in 3 interventions that are not widely implemented to date: prophylactic zinc supplementation, balanced energy-protein supplementation, and multiple micronutrient supplementation in pregnancy.

As these 2 studies point out, the treatment of childhood malnutrition and stunting may be costly and demanding, but outcomes will be worse if treated ineffectively, both on a personal basis and on a global scale.

Neurodevelopment, nutrition, and inflammation: the evolving global child health landscape

Bhutta ZA[1,2], Guerrant RL[3], Nelson CA[4–6]

[1]Centre for Global Child Health, The Hospital for Sick Children, Toronto, ON, Canada; [2]Centre of Excellence in Women and Child Health, Aga Khan University, Karachi, Pakistan; [3]Center for Global Health, Division of Infectious Diseases and International Health, University of Virginia School of Medicine, Charlottesville, VA, USA; [4]Laboratories of Cognitive Neuroscience, Boston Children's Hospital, Boston, MA, USA; [5]Department of Pediatrics, Harvard Medical School, Boston, MA, USA; [6]Human Development Program, Harvard Graduate School of Education, Cambridge, MA, USA

Pediatrics 2017;139(suppl 1):S12–S22

The last decade has witnessed major reductions in child mortality and a focus on saving lives with key interventions targeting major causes of child deaths, such as neonatal deaths and those due to childhood diarrhea and pneumonia. With the transition to Sustainable Development Goals, the global health community is expanding child health initiatives to address not only the ongoing need for reduced mortality, but also to decrease morbidity and adverse exposures toward improving health and developmental outcomes. The relationship between adverse environmental exposures frequently associated with factors operating in the pre-pregnancy period and during fetal development is well established. Also well appreciated are the developmental impacts (both short- and long-term) associated with postnatal factors, such as immunostimulation and environmental enteropathy, and the additional risks posed by the confluence of factors related to malnutrition, poor living conditions, and the high burden of infections. This article provides the pathogenesis and risk factors for adverse developmental outcomes among young children, setting the scene for potential interventions that can ameliorate these adversities among families and children at risk.

Comments A synthesis of current thinking relating prenatal factors includes epigenetic influences, with important postnatal environmental influences, immunostimulation and nutritional deficits with impaired growth and cognitive development. The review opens the possibility that while critical windows are important, there are opportunities for growth and especially developmental plasticity that goes well beyond the early years of life, opening the possibility of sustained interventions and investments in health, nutrition, and developmental strategies.

An individual-level meta-analysis assessing the impact of community-level sanitation access on child stunting, anemia, and diarrhea: evidence from DHS and MICS surveys

Larsen DA, Grisham T, Slawsky E, Narine L

Syracuse University Department of Public Health, Food Studies and Nutrition, Syracuse, NY, USA

PLoS Negl Trop Dis 2017;11:e0005591

Background: A lack of access to sanitation is an important risk factor in child health, facilitating fecal-oral transmission of pathogens including soil-transmitted helminthes and various causes of diarrheal disease. We conducted a meta-analysis of cross-sectional surveys to determine the impact that community-level sanitation access has on child health for children with and without household sanitation access.

Methodology: Using 301 2-stage demographic health surveys and multiple indicator cluster surveys conducted between 1990 and 2015, we calculated the sanitation access in the community as the proportion of households in the sampled cluster that had household access to any type of sanitation facility. We then conducted exact matching of children based on various predictors of living in a community with high access to sanitation. Using logistic regression with the matched group as a random intercept we examined the association between the child health outcomes of stunted growth, any anemia, moderate or severe anemia, and diarrhea in the previous 2 weeks and the exposure of living in a community with varying degrees of community-level sanitation access.

Results: For children with household-level sanitation access, living in a community with 100% sanitation access was associated with lowered odds of stunting (adjusted OR [AOR] 0.97, 95% CI 0.94–1.00; $n = 14,153$ matched groups, 1,175,167 children), any anemia (AOR 0.73; 95% CI 0.67–0.78; $n = 5,319$ matched groups, 299,033 children), moderate or severe anemia (AOR 0.72, 95% CI 0.68–0.77; $n = 5,319$ matched groups, 299,033 children), and diarrhea (AOR 0.94; 95% CI = 0.91–0.97); $n = 16,379$ matched groups, 1,603,731 children) compared to living in a community with <30% sanitation access. For children without household-level sanitation access, living in communities with 0% sanitation access was associated with higher odds of stunting (AOR 1.04, 95% CI 1.02–1.06; $n = 14,153$ matched groups, 1,175,167 children), any anemia (AOR 1.05, 95% CI 1.00–1.09; $n = 5,319$ matched groups, 299,033 children), moderate or severe anemia (AOR 1.04, 95% CI 1.00–1.09; $n = 5,319$ matched groups, 299,033 children) but not diarrhea (AOR 1.00, 95% CI 0.98–1.02; $n = 16,379$ matched groups, 1,603,731 children) compared to children without household-level sanitation access living in communities with 1–30% sanitation access.

Conclusions: Community-level sanitation access is associated with improved child health outcomes independent of household-level sanitation access. The proportion of children living in communities with 100% sanitation access throughout the world is appallingly low. Ensuring sanitation access to all by 2030 will greatly improve child health.

Comments This interesting analysis of available information in a range of demographic and health surveys corroborates initial findings from a similar analysis by Spears et al. [37] in India, and the findings from the Cochrane review of the relationship of water and sanitation interventions with childhood growth [38]. The finding that community-level sanitation status may impact linear growth and a range of health outcomes in children strongly supports the need to focus on such interventions alongside nutrition-sensitive interventions in populations.

References

1 UNICEF-WHO-The World Bank Group: Joint Child Malnutrition Estimates – Levels and Trends (2015 edition). Geneva, WHO, 2015. Available from: http://www.who.int/nutgrowthdb/estimates2014/en/ (cited April 21, 2016).

2 Haddad L, Achadi E, Bendech MA, Ahuja A, Bhatia K, Bhutta Z, Blösner M, Borghi E, Colecraft E, de Onis M, et al: The global nutrition report 2014: actions and accountability to accelerate the world's progress on nutrition. J Nutr 2015;145:663–671.

3 Lee SE, Stewart CP, Schulze KJ, Cole RN, Wu LS-F, Yager JD, Groopman JD, Khatry SK, Adhikari RK, Christian P, West KP Jr: The plasma proteome is associated with anthropometric status of undernourished nepalese school-aged children. J Nutr 2017; 147:304–313.

4 Rytter MJ, Namusoke H, Ritz C, Michaelsen KF, Briend A, Friis H, Dorthe Jeppesen D: Correlates of thymus size and changes during treatment of children with severe acute malnutrition: a cohort study. BMC Pediatr 2017;17:70.

5 McGrath CJ, Arndt MB, Walson JL: Biomarkers to stratify risk groups among children with malnutrition in resource-limited settings and to monitor response to intervention. Horm Res Paediatr 2017;88: 111–117.

6 Plovier H, Cani PD: Microbial impact on host metabolism: opportunities for novel treatments of nutritional disorders? Microbiol Spectr 2017;5:BAD-0002-2016.

7 Velly H, Britton RA, Preidis GA: Mechanisms of cross-talk between the diet, the intestinal microbiome, and the undernourished host. Gut Microbes 2017;8:98–112.

8 Dewey KG, Mridha MK, Matias SL, Arnold CD, Cummins JR, Khan MS, Maalouf-Manasseh Z, Siddiqui Z, Ullah MB, Vosti SA: Lipid-based nutrient supplementation in the first 1,000 days improves child growth in Bangladesh: a cluster-randomized effectiveness trial. Am J Clin Nutr 2017;105:944–957.

9 Iannotti LL, Lutter CK, Stewart CP, Gallegos Riofrío CA, Malo C, Reinhart G, Palacios A, Karp C, Chapnick M, Cox K, Waters WF: Eggs in early complementary feeding and child growth: a randomized controlled trial. Pediatrics 2017;140:e20163459.

10 Kureishy S, Khan GN, Arrif S, Ashraf K, Cespedes A, Habib MA, Hussain I, Ullah A, TurabA, Ahmed I, Zaida S, Soofi SB: A mixed method study to assess the effectiveness of food-based interventions to prevent stunting among children under-five years in Districts Thatta and Sujawal, Sindh Province, Pakistan: study protocol. BMC Public Health 2017;17:24.

11 Fatima S, Malkova D, Wright C, Gerasimidis K: Impact of therapeutic food compared to oral nutritional supplements on nutritional outcomes in mildly underweight healthy children in a low-medium-income society. Clin Nutr 2017;pii:S0261-5164(17)30097-3.

12 Baum JI, Miller JD, Gaines BL: The effect of egg supplementation on growth parameters in children participating in a school feeding program in rural Uganda: a pilot study. Food Nutr Res 2017;61:1330097.

13 Ganmaa D, Stuart JJ, Sumberzul N, Ninjin B, Giovannucci E, Kleinman K, Holick MF, Willett WC, Frazier LA, Rich-Edwards JW: Vitamin D supplementation and growth in urban Mongol school children: results from two randomized clinical trials. PLoS One 2017;12:e0175237.

14 Gat-Yablonski G, Yackobovitch-Gavan M, Phillip M: Which dietary components modulate longitudinal growth? Curr Opin Clin Nutr Metab Care 2017; 20:211–216.

15 Roberts JL, Stein AD: The impact of nutritional interventions beyond the first 2 years of life on linear growth: a systematic review and meta-analysis. Adv Nutr 2017;8:323–336.

16 McGovern ME, Krishna A, Aguayo VM, Subramanian SV: A review of the evidence linking child stunting to economic outcomes. Int J Epidemiol 2017;46: 1171–1191.

17 Shekar M, Kakietek J, D'Alimonte MR, Rogers HE, Eberwein JD Akuoku JK, Pereira P, Soe-Lin S, Hecht R: Reaching the global target to reduce stunting: an investment framework. Health Policy Plan 2017;32: 657–668.

18 Bhutta ZA, Guerrant RL, Nelson CA: Neurodevelopment, nutrition, and inflammation: the evolving global child health landscape. Pediatrics 2017; 139(suppl 1):S12–S22.

19 Larsen DA, Grisham T, Slawsky E, Narine L: An individual-level meta-analysis assessing the impact of community-level sanitation access on child stunting, anemia, and diarrhea: evidence from DHS and MICS surveys. PLoS Negl Trop Dis 2017;11:e0005591.

20 Chevalier P, Sevilla R, Zalles L, Sejas E, Belmonte G, Parent G: Study of thymus and thymocytes in Bolivian preschool children during recovery from severe acute malnutrition. J Nutr Immunol 1994;3:27–39.

21 Nassar MF, Younis NT, Tohamy AG, Dalam DM, El Badawy MA: T-lymphocyte subsets and thymic size in malnourished infants in Egypt: a hospital-based study. East Mediterr Health J 2007;13:1031–1042.

22 Rytter MJ, Babirekere-Iriso E, Namusoke H, Christensen VB, Michaelsen KF, Ritz C, Mortensen CG, Mupere E, Friis H: Risk factors for death in children during inpatient treatment of severe acute malnutrition: a prospective cohort study. Am J Clin Nutr 2017;105:494–502.

23 National Institute of Population Research and Training (NIPORT); Mitra and Associates; ICF International. Bangladesh Demographic and Health Survey 2014. Dhaka (Bangladesh), Rockville (MD): NIPORT, Mitra and Associates, and ICF International; 2016.

24 Lauritzen L, Carlson SE: Maternal fatty acid status during pregnancy and lactation and relation to newborn and infant status. Matern Child Nutr 2011; 7(suppl 2):41–58.

25 Makrides M, Collins CT, Gibson RA: Impact of fatty acid status on growth and neurobehavioural development in humans. Matern Child Nutr 2011;7(suppl 2):80–88.

26 Prentice AM, van der Merwe L: Impact of fatty acid status on immune function of children in low-income countries. Matern Child Nutr 2011;7(suppl 2):89–98.

27 Ijarotimi OS: Determinants of childhood malnutrition and consequences in developing countries. Curr Nutr Rep 2013;2:129–133.

28 Khan Y, Bhutta ZA: Nutritional deficiencies in the developing world: current status and opportunities for intervention. Pediatr Clin N Am 2010;57:1409–1441.

29 Dewey KG, Begum K: Long-term consequences of stunting in early life. Matern Child Nutr 2011;7(suppl 3):5–18.

30 Cao J, Wei X, Tang X, Jiang H, Fan Z, Yu Q, Chen J, Liu Y, Li T: Effects of egg and vitamin A supplementation on hemoglobin, retinol status and physical growth levels of primary and middle school students in Chongqing, China. Asia Pac J Clin Nutr 2013;22:214–221.

31 Sudfeld CR, Manji KP, Smith ER, Aboud S, Kisenge R, Fawzi WW, Duggan CP: Vitamin D deficiency Is not associated with growth or the incidence of common morbidities among tanzanian infants. J Pediatr Gastroenterol Nutr 2017;65:467–474.

32 Veena SR, Krishnaveni GV, Srinivasan K, Thajna KP, Hegde BG, Gale CR, Fall CH: Association between maternal vitamin D status during pregnancy and offspring cognitive function during childhood and adolescence. Asia Pac J Clin Nutr 2017;26:438–449.

33 Darling AL, Rayman MP, Steer CD, Golding J, Lanham-New SA, Bath SC: Association between maternal vitamin D status in pregnancy and neurodevelopmental outcomes in childhood: results from the Avon Longitudinal Study of Parents and Children (ALSPAC). Br J Nutr 2017;117:1682–1692.

34 Chowdhury R, Taneja S, Bhandari N, Sinha B, Upadhyay RP, Bhan MK, Strand TA: Vitamin-D deficiency predicts infections in young north Indian children: a secondary data analysis. PLoS One 2017; 12:e0170509.

35 Lundeen EA, Behrman JR, Crookston BT, Dearden KA, Engle P, Georgiadis A, Penny ME, Stein AD: Growth faltering and recovery in children aged 1–8 years in four low- and middle-income countries: young Lives. Public Health Nutr 2014;17:2131–2137.

36 Prentice AM, Ward KA, Goldberg GR, Jarjou LM, Moore SE, Fulford AJ, Prentice A: Critical windows for nutritional interventions against stunting. Am J Clin Nutr 2013;97:911–918.

37 Spears D, Ghosh A, Cumming O: Open defecation and childhood stunting in India: an ecological analysis of new data from 112 districts. PLoS One 2013; 8:e73784.

38 Dangour AD, Watson L, Cumming O, Boisson S, Che Y, Velleman Y, Cavill S, Allen E, Uauy R: Interventions to improve water quality and supply, sanitation and hygiene practices, and their effects on the nutritional status of children. Cochrane Database Syst Rev 2013;(8):CD009382.

Koletzko B, Shamir R, Turck D, Phillip M (eds): Nutrition and Growth: Yearbook 2018.
World Rev Nutr Diet. Basel, Karger, 2018, vol 117, pp 151–164 (DOI: 10.1159/000484504)

Pregnancy: Impact of Maternal Nutrition on Intrauterine Fetal Growth

Liran Hiersch[1,2] · Yariv Yogev[1,2]

[1]Department of Obstetrics and Gynecology, Lis Maternity Hospital, Sourasky Medical Center, and
[2]Sackler Faculty of Medicine, Tel Aviv University, Tel Aviv, Israel

This chapter of the YEARBOOK on NUTRITION AND GROWTH reviews important articles published between July 2016 and June 2017 concerning the impact of maternal nutrition during pregnancy on intrauterine fetal growth. We carefully selected human studies, mainly of randomized controlled or prospective design, along with several animal studies dealing with the effect of several nutrient supplementations on fetal growth and metabolic programming. This year, we focused on studies addressing the issue of fetal adiposity and maternal nutrition during pregnancy that may affect this outcome. Hopefully, this chapter will aid clinicians to update their knowledge on the effect of various intervention options and their effect on fetal growth and development.

Key articles reviewed for this chapter

Human Studies

Maternal dietary intake during pregnancy and offspring body composition: The Healthy Start Study

Crume TL, Brinton JT, Shapiro A, Kaar J, Glueck DH, Siega-Riz AM, Dabelea D

Am J Obstet Gynecol 2016;215:609.e1–e8

Maternal macronutrient intake during pregnancy is associated with neonatal abdominal adiposity: the Growing Up in Singapore Towards healthy Outcomes (GUSTO) study

Chen LW, Tint MT, Fortier MV, Aris IM, Bernard JY, Colega M, Gluckman PD, Saw SM, Chong YS, Yap F, Godfrey KM, Kramer MS, van Dam RM, Chong MF, Lee YS

J Nutr 2016;146:1571–1579

Animal Studies

The early infant gut microbiome varies in association with a maternal high-fat diet

Chu DM, Antony KM, Ma J, Prince AL, Showalter L, Moller M, Aagaard KM

Genome Med 2016;8:77

Maternal blood lipid profile during pregnancy and associations with child adiposity: findings from the ROLO study

Geraghty AA, Alberdi G, O'Sullivan EJ, O'Brien EC, Crosbie B, Twomey PJ, McAuliffe FM

PLoS One 11:e0161206

Maternal diet quality in pregnancy and neonatal adiposity: the Healthy Start Study

Shapiro AL, Kaar JL, Crume TL, Starling AP, Siega-Riz AM, Ringham BM, Glueck DH, Norris JM, Barbour LA, Friedman JE, Dabelea D

Int J Obes 2016;40:1056–1062

Association of prenatal lipid-based nutritional supplementation with fetal growth in rural Gambia

Johnson W, Darboe MK, Sosseh F, Nshe P, Prentice AM, Moore SE

Matern Child Nutr 2017;13:e12367

The relationship between 25-hydroxyvitamin D concentration in early pregnancy and pregnancy outcomes in a large, prospective cohort

Boyle VT, Thorstensen EB, Mourath D, Jones MB, McCowan LM, Kenny LC, Baker PN. Baker on behalf of the SCOPE Consortium

Br J Nutr 2016;116:1409–1415

The effect of maternal nutrition level during the periconception period on fetal muscle development and plasma hormone concentrations in sheep

Sen U, Sirin E, Yildiz S, Aksoy Y, Ulutas Z, Kuran M

Animal 2016;10:1689 1696

Maternal consumption of low isoflavone soy protein isolate alters hepatic gene
expression and liver development in rat offspring

Won SB, Han A, Kwon YH

J Nutr Biochem 2017;42:51–61

Human Studies

Maternal dietary intake during pregnancy and offspring body composition: the Healthy Start Study

Crume TL[1], Brinton JT[2], Shapiro A[3], Kaar J[4], Glueck DH[2], Siega-Riz AM[5], Dabelea D[3]

[1]Department of Epidemiology, Colorado School of Public Health, University of Colorado-Denver Anschutz Medical Center, Denver, CO, USA; [2]Department of Biostatistics and Informatics, Colorado School of Public Health, University of Colorado-Denver Anschutz Medical Center, Denver, CO, USA; [3]Department of Epidemiology, Colorado School of Public Health, University of Colorado-Denver Anschutz Medical Center, Denver, CO., USA; [4]Department of Pediatrics and Nutrition, School of Medicine, University of Colorado-Denver Anschutz Medical Center, Denver, CO, USA; [5]Departments of Epidemiology and Nutrition, Gillings School of Global Public Health, University of North Carolina at Chapel Hill, Chapel Hill, NC, USA

Am J Obstet Gynecol 2016;215:609.e1–e8

Background: Animal models suggest that maternal dietary intake during pregnancy can affect the infant body composition. However, studies involving human population are lacking.

Aims: The current study aimed to explore the influence of maternal macronutrient intake and balance during pregnancy on neonatal body size and composition, including fat mass and fat-free mass.

Methods: This is an analysis of 1,040 mother-offspring pairs enrolled in a prospective observational cohort: the Healthy Start Study. Maternal diet during pregnancy was collected using dietary recalls (up to 8). Neonatal body composition was directly measured using air displacement plethysmography. Usual dietary intake during pregnancy was estimated using the National Cancer Institute measurement error model. The associations between maternal dietary intake and neonatal body composition were investigated by using multivariable partition (nonisocaloric) and nutrient density (isocaloric) linear regression models.

Results: The median macronutrient composition during pregnancy was 32.2% from fat, 15.0% from protein, and 47.8% from carbohydrates. In the partition multivariate regression model, no association was found between individual macronutrient intake values and neonatal birth weight or fat-free mass (FFM). However, an association was found between individual macronutrient and fat mass. About 418 kJ increases in total fat, saturated fat, unsaturated fat, and total carbohydrates were associated with 4.2 g ($p = 0.03$), 11.1 g ($p = 0.003$), 5.9 g ($p = 0.04$), and 2.9 g ($p = 0.02$) increase in neonatal fat mass, respectively. This increase was independent of maternal pre-pregnancy body mass index (BMI). In the nutrient density multivariate regression model, macronutrient balance was not associated with neonatal FFM, fat mass or birth weight after adjustment for pre-pregnancy BMI.

Conclusions: Increase in maternal intake of total fat, saturated fat, unsaturated fat, and total carbohydrates is associated with an increase in neonatal adiposity.

Comment   The association between maternal dietary intake during pregnancy and neonatal body composition is interesting and was mainly demonstrated in animal models. The relationship between maternal consumption of high-fat diet during pregnancy and the change in the offspring adiposity was previously demonstrated in rodent and other species. In contrast, human studies are less conclusive. Moreover, they are more prone to substantial methodological limitations as most studies of pregnant women have relied on food frequency questionnaires, which are prone to measurement error and are biased by patient self-reporting.

The clinical relevance of the findings of the current studies is several-fold. First, it is suggested that total energy intake sources contribute more than the calorie source as this study found that neonatal fat mass was influenced by various maternal macronutrients intake. Second, it is important to note that the magnitude of effect is small as a 418 kJ increase from saturated fatty acid is associated with only an 11.1 g or 4% increase in fat mass at birth. Yet, this increase is independent of maternal pre-pregnancy BMI, which is known to be correlated with neonatal adiposity. Third, this study provides evidence that the effect of maternal energy intake during pregnancy mainly affects the neonatal fat mass and had no detectable influence on FFM or even neonatal birth weight. The results of the study are important as they suggest potential nutritional interventions during pregnancy for the reduction of neonatal adiposity, without altering the overall neonatal body size or lean mass.

Maternal macronutrient intake during pregnancy is associated with neonatal abdominal adiposity: the Growing Up in Singapore Towards healthy Outcomes (GUSTO) study

Chen LW[1], Tint MT[2], Fortier MV[5], Aris IM[7], Bernard JY[7], Colega M[7], Gluckman PD[7,8], Saw SM[4], Chong YS[2,7], Yap F[6,9], Godfrey KM[10], Kramer MS[2,11], van Dam RM[3,4,12], Chong MF[4,7,13] Lee YS[1,7,14]

[1]Department of Paediatrics, [2]Department of Obstetrics and Gynaecology, [3]Department of Medicine, Yong Loo Lin School of Medicine, [4]Saw Swee Hock School of Public Health, National University of Singapore, Singapore; [5]Department of Diagnostic and Interventional Imaging and [6]Department of Pediatric Endocrinology, KK Women's and Children's Hospital, Singapore; [7]Singapore Institute for Clinical Sciences, Agency for Science, Technology, and Research, Singapore; [8]Liggins Institute, University of Auckland, Auckland, New Zealand; [9]Duke–NUS Graduate Medical School, Lee Kong Chian School of Medicine, Singapore; [10]MRC Lifecourse Epidemiology Unit and NIHR Southampton Biomedical Research Centre, University of Southampton and University Hospital Southampton NHS Foundation Trust, Southampton, UK; [11]Departments of Pediatrics and Epidemiology, Biostatistics, and Occupational Health, McGill University Faculty of Medicine, Montreal, Canada; [12]Department of Nutrition, Harvard School of Public Health, Boston, MA, USA; [13]Clinical Nutrition Research Centre, Singapore Institute for Clinical Sciences, A*STAR, Singapore; [14]Khoo Teck Puat–National University Children's Medical Institute, National University Health System, Singapore

J Nutr 2016;146:1571–1579

Background: The body composition of infant was found to be associated with the risk for metabolic dysregulation later in life. However, not many have examined that the maternal macronutrient intake may attenuate the neonatal body composition. Moreover, in most of the prior studies, a proxy measure of body composition was used, which may not reflect body fat distribution, particularly abdominal internal adiposity.

Aims: To investigate the influence of maternal macronutrient intake on neonatal abdominal adiposity measured in a multi-ethnic Asian mother-offspring cohort.

Methods: The current analysis includes 320 mother-offspring dyads with complete macronutrient intake and adiposity information. Maternal macronutrient intake was ascertained using a 24-h dietary recall at 26–28 weeks gestation. Neonatal abdominal adiposity was assessed using magnetic resonance imaging (MRI) in the second week of life. Associations were assessed by both substitution and addition models using multivariable linear regressions.

Results: The mean maternal age was 30 years. Maternal ethnicity diversity was as follows: 44% Chinese, 38% Malay, and 18% Indians. Mothers consumed $15.5 \pm 4.3\%$ (mean $\pm$ SD) of their energy intakes from protein, $32.4 \pm 7.7\%$ from fat, and $52.1 \pm 9.0\%$ from carbohydrate. A lower carbohydrate/fat higher protein diet during pregnancy was associated with lower neonatal abdominal internal adipose tissue (IAT; β [95% CI] –0.18 [–0.35 to –0.001] mL per 1% protein to carbohydrate substitution and –0.25 [–0.46 to –0.04] mL per 1% protein to fat substitution). These findings were more pronounced in males than in females (P-interactions <0.05). Higher maternal intake of animal protein (–0.26 [–0.47 to –0.05] mL for fat substitution), but not plant protein, was associated with lower offspring IAT. In contrast, maternal macronutrient intake was not consistently associated with infant anthropometric measurements, including abdominal circumference and subscapular skinfold thickness.

Conclusions: Increased maternal protein intake (as opposed to fat or carbohydrates) at 26–28 weeks of gestation was associated with lower abdominal internal adiposity in the offspring.

Comment   The rate of obesity in children and adulthood is rising and becoming a true epidemic in both developed and developing countries. Although overall adiposity is related to metabolic complication including hypertension and diabetes, many studies have reported that patients with increased visceral adipose tissue (intra-abdominal fat surrounding the internal organs) are at risk in particular. This may be due to the fact that adipocytes from visceral adipose tissue are more metabolically active and insulin-resistant compared with adipocytes from subcutaneous adipose tissue.

In this Asian multi-ethnic mother-offspring cohort study, higher maternal protein intake at the expense of carbohydrate or fat intake was associated with lower abdominal IAT in the newborns. The use of MRI for the assessment of visceral adiposity is a significant strength of this study as MRI is considered the gold standard method for this purpose. Another important point to consider in reviewing this study is that neonatal gender and maternal ethnicity modified the associations between maternal macronutrient intake and neonatal abdominal adiposity. The association of higher maternal protein intake and lower offspring IAT was stronger in boys.

Overall, the results of the study are important as optimizing maternal dietary balance during pregnancy might be a new approach to potentially improve the offspring body composition. Moreover, the traditional tools for the assessment of adiposity in the offspring are birth weight and anthropometric index. The lack of association between maternal macronutrient intake and various proxy measures of adiposity at birth indicated that accurate body fat distribution measurement early in life may provide more valuable insights on the risk for metabolic abnormalities.

The early infant gut microbiome varies in association with a maternal high-fat diet

Chu DM[1–3], Antony KM[1], Ma J[1], Prince AL[1], Showalter L[1], Moller M[1] and Aagaard KM[1–5]

[1]Department of Obstetrics and Gynecology, Baylor College of Medicine, Houston, TX, USA; [2]Interdepartmental Program in Translational Biology and Molecular Medicine, Baylor College of Medicine, Houston, TX, USA; [3]Medical Scientist Training Program, Baylor College of Medicine, Houston, TX, USA; [4]Departments of Molecular and Human Genetics, Molecular and Cell Biology, and Molecular Physiology and Biophysics, Baylor College of Medicine, Houston, TX, USA; [5]Division of Maternal-Fetal Medicine, Baylor College of Medicine, Houston, TX, USA

Genome Med 2016;8:77

Background: Despite traditional presumption, emerging evidence suggests that the in utero environment is not sterile. Animal studies demonstrated transmission of commensal bacteria from mother to fetus during gestation, though it is unclear what modulates this process. In humans, maternal high-fat diet during pregnancy and lactation was previously found to persistently shape the juvenile gut microbiome.

Aims: This study aimed to interrogate whether a maternal high-fat diet similarly alters the neonatal and infant gut microbiome in early life in a population-based human longitudinal cohort.

Methods: A prospective cohort study of 163 women enrolling either in the early third trimester or intrapartum was used. Of them, 81 have consented to longitudinal sampling through the postpartum period. Samples were collected from multiple body sites of the neonates at delivery and by 6 weeks of age, including stool and meconium. Maternal nutrition over the past month prior to sample collection was assessed using a rapid dietary questionnaire to estimate intake of fat, added sugars, and fiber (National Health and Examination Survey). DNA was extracted from each infant meconium/stool sample (MoBio) and subjected to 16S rRNA gene sequencing and analysis.

Results: Maternal fat dietary intake ranged from 14.0 to 55.2%, with mean values of 33.1 ± 6.1%. Mothers whose diets significantly differed from the mean (±1 SD) were divided into two distinct groups: the control group ($n = 13$, $\mu = 24.4\%$) and a high-fat group ($n = 13$, $\mu = 43.1$). Neonatal stool (meconium) analysis revealed differently clustered microbiome between the groups. Linear effect size (LEfSe) feature selection identified several taxa that discriminated the groups. Relative depletion of bacteroides was noticed in the group of neonates exposed to a maternal high-fat gestational diet, which persisted for 6 weeks of age.

Conclusions: Independent of maternal BMI, a maternal high-fat diet is associated with distinct changes in the neonatal gut microbiome at birth and even at 4–6 weeks of age. These findings highlight the importance of counseling pregnant mothers on macronutrient consumption during gestation and lactation.

Comment   The human microbiome encompasses a rich ecosystem of approximately 90 trillion microbes that aid in human metabolism and impact host physiology. It was previously found that microbiota is associated with the presence of obesity, inflammatory bowel disease, and autoimmune disease. In contrast to prior beliefs that the in-utero environment is sterile, recent data indicate that microbiota are present in the placenta and amniotic fluid of healthy, term pregnancies without any clinical evidence of infection. The findings of this study are important since not only the neonatal gut microbiome immediately after delivery revealed that it varied by virtue of maternal gestational diet, but also that this variation persisted for several weeks after birth. In the neonates of the maternal high-fat diet groups a relative depletion of bacteroides species in this early time period was found. This depletion may influence the infant's future risk of developing obesity. Yet, the literature to date is controversial regarding the association of bacteroides species and obesity, so whether such effect would be protective or contributory is unknown. It is important to note that maternal diet in the postpartum period was not explored in this study. Therefore, the effect of maternal diet and breast milk composition on the results regarding neonatal microbiome at 4–6 weeks of life cannot be assessed and may bias the results.

Although clear guidelines have been established for specific micronutrient and total caloric intake during gestation and lactation, the recommendations for macronutrients, including processed sugars, fats, and fibers are less. These findings, if proven in other large studies, may warrant consideration for refining dietary recommendations during pregnancy.

Maternal blood lipid profile during pregnancy and associations with child adiposity: findings from the ROLO study

Geraghty AA[1], Alberdi G[1], O'Sullivan EJ[1], O'Brien EC[1], Crosbie B[2], Twomey PJ[2, 3], McAuliffe FM[1]

[1]UCD Obstetrics and Gynaecology, School of Medicine, University College Dublin, National Maternity Hospital, Dublin, Ireland; [2]Clinical Chemistry, St. Vincent's University Hospital, Dublin, Ireland; [3]UCD School of Medicine, University College Dublin, Dublin, Ireland

PLoS One 2016;11:e0161206

Background: It is well established that the in-utero environment affects fetal growth. Research concerning maternal hyperlipidemia has shown a relation with fetal growth mainly in women with hyperglycemia. However, this relationship in euglycemic women is scarce.

Aims: This study aimed to examine the relationship between maternal blood lipid profile and infant adiposity up to 2 years of age.

Methods: The ROLO (Randomized control trial of Low glycemic index diet vs. no dietary intervention in pregnancy to prevent recurrence of a large baby) study is a randomized trial that was conducted in Ireland in to assess whether low glycemic index in women with prior macrosomic infant may modulate the birth weight. In the current study, only data from 331 mother-child pairs were analyzed. Maternal dietary intakes were recorded and fasting blood lipids, leptin, and homeostatic model assessment index were measured in early and late pregnancy and cord blood. Infant anthropometric measurements and skinfold thicknesses were recorded at birth, 6 months and 2 years. Correlation and regression analyses were used to explore associations between maternal blood lipid status and infant adiposity.

Results: A significant increase in all maternal blood lipids during pregnancy was shown. Maternal dietary fat intake was positively associated with total cholesterol levels in early pregnancy. Late pregnancy triglycerides were positively associated with birth weight ($p = 0.03$), while cord blood triglycerides were negatively associated with birth weight ($p = 0.01$). Cord high-density lipoprotein cholesterol (HDL-C) was negatively associated with infant weight at 6 months ($p = 0.005$). No other maternal blood lipids were associated with infant weight or adiposity up to 2 years of age.

Conclusions: An association was found between maternal and fetal triglycerides and birth weight. Cord HDL-C was found to be associated with weight at 6 months. Thus, maternal lipid concentrations may exert in-utero influences on infant body composition.

Comment   The rate of childhood obesity is increasing, with the World Health Organization estimating that over 41 million children aged under 5 years are obese. Obese children are at increased risk for metabolic-related morbidity later in life, including type 2 diabetes, cardiovascular disease, and metabolic syndrome. Therefore, studies focusing on understanding variables associated with childhood obesity are of most importance, particularly those addressing the association between maternal diet during pregnancy and the child's body composition.

The current study is important, mainly because it is one of few prospective studies to have both maternal and fetal blood samples on multiple occasions during pregnancy, along with detailed infant anthropometry up to the age of 2 years. It demonstrated that dietary intakes of fat in early pregnancy were associated with total maternal cholesterol concentrations. In addition, it demonstrated that the concentrations of all blood lipids increased significantly as pregnancy progressed. Although these issues were previously studied, the current study adds to the current knowledge of associations between maternal blood lipid concentrations during pregnancy and outcomes for the baby. In addition, the finding regarding the association of higher HDL-C concentrations in cord blood and lower infant weight at 6 months was not previously reported. As maternal diet during pregnancy is modifiable, this represents a way to potentially reduce childhood obesity levels. Yet, it is important to remember that the cohort of the ROLO study was a high-risk group for macrosomia and further research should be conducted before official recommendation can be made in the general obstetric population.

Maternal diet quality in pregnancy and neonatal adiposity: the Healthy Start Study

Shapiro AL[1], Kaar JL[2], Crume TL[1], Starling AP[1], Siega-Riz AM[3], Ringham BM[4], Glueck DH[4], Norris JM[1], Barbour LA[5], Friedman JE[6], Dabelea D[1]

[1]Department of Epidemiology, Colorado School of Public Health (CSPH), Aurora, CO, USA; [2]Division of Pediatric Nutrition, University of Colorado School of Medicine, Aurora, CO, USA; [3]Departments of Epidemiology and Nutrition, Gillings School of Global Public Health, University of North Carolina at Chapel Hill, Chapel Hill, NC, USA; [4]Department of Biostatistics and Informatics, CSPH, Aurora, CO, USA; [5]Division of Endocrinology, Metabolism and Diabetes, Department of Medicine University of Colorado, Denver, CO, USA; [6]Departments of Pediatrics and Biochemistry and Molecular Genetics, School of Medicine, University of Colorado, Denver, CO, USA

Int J Obes 2016;40:1056–1062

Background: Maternal diet in pregnancy can influence fetal growth and development.

Aims: To test the hypothesis concerning an association between poor maternal diet quality during pregnancy and increase in neonatal adiposity (percent fat mass [%FM]) at birth.

Methods: An observational cohort of 1,079 mother-offspring pairs was used. For each woman, Healthy Eating Index-2010 (HEI-2010) scores were calculated according to maternal diet, which was assessed via repeated Automated Self-Administered 24-h dietary recalls. The scores in the HEI-2010 was dichotomized into scores of ≤57 and >57. Lower scores represented poorer diet quality. Within 72 h after delivery, neonatal %FM was assessed using air displacement plethysmography. The relationship between maternal diet quality and neonatal %FM, FM, and fat-free mass were explored while adjusting for potential confounders including pre-pregnancy BMI, physical activity, maternal age, smoking status, energy intake, hypertensive disorders during pregnancy, infant sex, and gestational age at delivery.

Hiersch · Yogev

Results: The total HEI-2010 score ranged between 18.2 and 89.5 (mean: 54.2, SD 13.6). An HEI-2010 score of ≤57 was significantly associated with higher neonatal %FM ($\beta = 0.58$, 95% CI 0.07–1.1, $p < 0.05$) and FM ($\beta = 20.74$; 95% CI 1.49–40.0; $p < 0.05$) but no difference in fat-free mass was observed.

Conclusions: Neonatal adiposity is increased in cases of poor maternal diet quality during pregnancy independent of maternal pre-pregnancy BMI and total caloric intake.

Comment   Maternal obesity was found to be associated with increased birth weight and neonatal adiposity in large prospective cohort studies. In turn, these offsprings are at greater risk for childhood obesity and future metabolic dysregulation. Unfortunately, it is challenging to implement interventions that can successfully help women to maintain proper weight before becoming pregnant, partly because a significant portion of pregnancies are unplanned. Therefore, research should be shifted from reducing maternal weight before and during pregnancy to other interventions that may also affect fetal overgrowth and offspring adiposity, including the improvement of maternal diet and nutrition. The present analysis aimed to fill this information gap using the Healthy Start cohort, a pre-birth, multi-ethnic cohort of 1,410 mother-offspring pairs. The importance of this study lies in the fact that while maternal nutrition during pregnancy has been previously studied in relation to birth outcomes, this study focuses on the effect of maternal diet quality during pregnancy on neonatal body composition, which was scarcely studied before. The researchers demonstrated that lower maternal diet quality has a significant impact on neonatal adiposity, irrespective of maternal pre-pregnancy BMI. Of note, neonates of women with lower diet quality had a mean increase of 24.9 g of fat mass, compared with those whose mothers had a higher diet quality. In comparison, the mean effect of maternal obesity on neonatal fat mas was 47.5 g (obese vs. normal weight mothers). This finding highlights the magnitude of diet quality among other effectors of fetal and neonatal adiposity and the potential importance of dietary interventions during pregnancy.

Association of prenatal lipid–based nutritional supplementation with fetal growth in rural Gambia

Johnson W[1], Darboe MK[2], Sosseh F[2], Nshe P[2], Prentice AM[2], Moore SE[1]

[1]MRC Human Nutrition Research, Cambridge, UK; [2]MRC International Nutrition Group, MRC, Unit The Gambia, Fajara, Banjul, The Gambia

Matern Child Nutr 2017;13:e12367

Background: Prenatal supplementation with protein-energy (PE) and/or multiple-micronutrients (MMNs) may improve fetal growth, however, inconsistent evidence exists regarding lipid-based nutritional supplements (LNS) and its relation to fetal growth.

Aims: The aim of the study was to explore the association between LNS during pregnancy and fetal growth, and explore how efficacy varies depending on the nutritional status.

Methods: A post-hoc analysis of non-primary outcomes in a trial in Gambia was conducted. Pregnant women ($n = 620$) were individually randomized, into 4 arms: (a) iron and folic acid tablet (usual care, referent group), (b) MMNs tablet, (c) PE + LNS, and (d) PE + LNS + MMNs tablet. Analysis of variance examined unadjusted differences in fetal biometry z-scores at 20 and 30 weeks and neonatal anthropometry z-scores, while regression tested for modification of intervention-outcome associations by season and maternal characteristics including maternal height, BMI, and weight gain during pregnancy.

Results: Z-scores at birth were not greater in the intervention arms than the FeFol arm (e.g., birth weight z-scores: FeFol –0.71, MMN –0.63, PE –0.64, PE + MMN –0.62; group-wise p = 0.796). In regression analyses, intervention associations with birthweight and head circumference were modified by maternal weight gain between booking and 30 weeks gestation (e.g., PE + MMN associations with birth weight were +0.462 z-scores (95% CI 0.097–0.826) in the highest quartile of weight gain but –0.099 z-scores (–0.459 to 0.260) in the lowest).

Conclusion: No strong evidence was found regarding the use of prenatal LNS and improvement in fetal growth in the study sample. However, some improvement was noticed in the subgroup of women who had the highest weight gain.

Comments   It is estimated that almost half of pediatric mortality is related to undernutrition in the developing counties, with fetal growth restriction alone accounting for 12% of deaths. It was hypothesized that a balanced prenatal protein-energy (PE) and MMN supplementation could potentially reduce fetal growth restriction and that the impact may be best observed in women who are more nutritionally vulnerable, like in rural Gambia. Although the results of the current study failed to demonstrate any association between prenatal LNS intervention and better fetal growth in the whole sample, it was found to have an additional value in the subgroup of women who demonstrated the greatest gestational weight gain. It implies that prenatal LNS intervention cannot be a substitution for a balanced diet and for proper nutrition during pregnancy and that we need to take all efforts to make sure that women will have proper diet and will be well-nourished especially during the pregnancy period. Only after we accomplish this objective, will we add interventions, like LNS, to improve fetal growth.

The relationship between 25-hydroxyvitamin D concentration in early pregnancy and pregnancy outcomes in a large, prospective cohort

Boyle VT[1], Thorstensen EB[1], Mourath D[2], Jones MB[3], McCowan LME[4], Kenny LC [5] and Baker PN[1, 6] on behalf of the SCOPE Consortium

[1]Gravida: National Centre for Growth and Development, The Liggins Institute, The University of Auckland, Auckland, New Zealand; [2]Medical Program, Linköping University, Linköping, Sweden; [3]Institute of Natural and Mathematical Sciences, Massey University, New Zealand; [4]The Department of Obstetrics and Gynaecology, South Auckland Clinical School, The University of Auckland, Auckland, New Zealand; [5]The Irish Centre for Fetal and Neonatal Translational Research (INFANT) and the Department of Obstetrics and Gynaecology, University College Cork, Cork, Ireland; [6]The College of Medicine, Biological Sciences and Psychology, University of Leicester, Leicester LE1 7RH, UK

Br J Nutr 2016;116:1409–1415

Background: Low plasma vitamin D levels have been associated with an increased rate of complications in pregnancy. Controversy remains as findings have been inconsistent between disparate populations.

Aims: The aim of the current study was to explore the association between vitamin D status and the risk for adverse pregnancy outcomes.

Methods: A large, prospective cohort study was conducted. Maternal 25-Hydroxyvitamin D concentration in serum samples collected at 15 weeks of gestation from 1,710 New Zealand women was analyzed. The associations between vitamin D status and pre-eclampsia, preterm birth, small for gestational age (SGA), and gestational diabetes were investigated.

Results: The mean vitamin D level was 72.9 nmol/L. Overall, only 23% had 25-hydroxyvitamin D concentrations <50 nmol/L, and 5% of women had concentrations <25 nmol/L. Those with vitamin D concentrations <75 nmol/L at 15 weeks of gestation were at increased risk for gestational diabetes mellitus than those with concentrations >75 nmol/L (OR 2.3; 95% CI 1.1–5.1). This effect was not significant when adjustments were made for BMI and ethnicity. No increased risk was found regarding the risk for preeclampsia, preterm birth or SGA infants.

Conclusion: In this vitamin D-replete pregnancy cohort, 25-hydroxyvitamin D concentration at 15 weeks of gestation did not predict pregnancy outcomes including preeclampsia, SGA, spontaneous preterm birth, and GDM when adjustments were made for confounders.

Comments   There is a controversy in the literature regarding the vitamin D supplementation during pregnancy. Some studies, including a recently published meta-analysis [1] found no difference in the rate of SGA or low birth weight with vitamin D supplementation in pregnancy. However, another systemic review on vitamin D supplementation in pregnancy found a reduced incidence of preeclampsia, preterm birth, and low birth weight (<2,500 *g*) [2]. In this prospective study, maternal vitamin D levels were not found to be associated with pregnancy-related complications. The execution of studies exploring the association between vitamin D levels and birth weight among other complication is not easy. There are many etiologies for reduced birth weight and controlling for potential confounders is not an easy task. Moreover, it is important to notice that vitamin D status in the population itself (vitamin D replete vs. deplete population) may also affect the results in studies addressing the added value of vitamin D supplementation. In addition, vitamin D may be a surrogate marker for other causative factors that vary between populations, particularly those with seasonal variation. Finally, the ethnic group studied may also affect the results since genetic polymorphisms of the vitamin D nuclear receptor and vitamin D binding protein exists.

The most important take home message from the current study is to understand its setting and methods and to be cautious in translating the results to other populations.

The effect of maternal nutrition level during the periconception period on fetal muscle development and plasma hormone concentrations in sheep

Sen U[1], Sirin E[1], Yildiz S[2], Aksoy Y[3], Ulutas Z[4], Kuran M[5]

[1]Department of Agricultural Biotechnology, Faculty of Agriculture, Ahi Evran University, Asikpasa, Kirsehir, Turkey; [2]Department of Physiology, Faculty of Medicine, Inonu University, Malatya, Turkey; [3]Department of Animal Science, Faculty of Agriculture, Osmangazi University, Eskisehir, Turkey; [4]Department of Animal Production and Technologies, Ayhan Sahenk Faculty of Agriculture Science and Technologies, Nigde University, Nigde, Turkey; [5]Department of Agricultural Biotechnology, Faculty of Agriculture, Ondokuz Mayis University, Atakum, Samsun, Turkey

Animal 2016;10:1689–1696

Background: Maternal malnutrition during gestation may alter fetal growth, and newborn's growth and development.

Aims: To examine the association between maternal nutrition during the periconception period and the muscle development of fetus and maternal-fetal plasma hormone concentrations in sheep.

Methods: Estrus was synchronized in 55 Karayaka ewes and were either fed ad libitum (well-fed [WF], $n = 23$) or 0.5× maintenance (under-fed [UF], $n = 32$) 6 days before and 7 days after mating. Those who did not become pregnant and ewes carrying twins and female fetuses were excluded from the study. Singleton male fetuses from WF ($n = 8$) and UF ($n = 5$) ewes were collected on day 90 of gestation and placental characteristics, fetal birth weight and dimensions, fetal organs and muscles weights were recorded. Maternal and fetal blood samples were collected on day 7 after mating and on day 90 of pregnancy, respectively, and plasma hormone concentrations were analyzed.

Results: Maternal nutrition during the periconception period had no statistically significant effect on placental characteristics, birth weight and dimensions, organs and muscles weights of the fetuses. In addition, maternal intake did not affect fiber numbers and the muscle cross-sectional area of the fetal longissimus dorsi (LD), semitendinosus (ST) muscles, but the cross-sectional area of the secondary fibers in the fetal LD and ST muscles from the UF ewes were higher than those from the WF ewes ($p < 0.05$). Moreover, a lower ratio of secondary to primary fibers in the ST muscle was tended in fetuses from the UF ewes. Regarding plasma concentration of hormones, no significant changes in fetal plasma insulin and maternal and fetal plasma IGF-I, cortisol, progesterone, free T3 and T4 concentrations were noted between the groups. However, maternal cortisol concentrations were lower while insulin concentrations were higher in the WF ewes than those in the UF ewes.

Conclusions: In lambs, reduced maternal feed intake during the periconception period may alter muscle fiber diameter without affecting fiber types, fetal weights and organ developments and plasma hormone concentrations in fetus.

Comment Maternal undernutrition during gestation not only affects nutrient and hormone concentrations in blood, but may also change the intrauterine micro-environment. This in turn may affect placental-fetal development, and therefore, influence subsequent development of the offspring. In addition, maternal endocrine status was previously shown to be affected by maternal nutrition level during the periconception period. The findings of the current study suggest that low nutrient intake during the periconception period affect the cross-sectional area of secondary fibers (in LD and ST muscles) and changes the ratio of secondary to primary fibers (in ST muscle). Of note, despite these effects, no changes were observed regarding fetal weights, placental characteristics, fetal organ developments, and fetal plasma hormone concentrations. These findings are important since these microscopic changes may go unnoticed when only clinical parameters such as birth weight are studied. These results teach us to explore microscopic effects that may have long-term outcomes and not only focus on the obvious outcome measures. Future studies may explain the underlying mechanisms involved in early embryonic development and programming of the muscle cell lineage.

Maternal consumption of low isoflavone soy protein isolate alters hepatic gene expression and liver development in rat offspring

Won SB[1], Han A[1], Kwon YH[2]

[1]Department of Food and Nutrition, Seoul National University, Seoul, Republic of Korea; [2]Research Institute of Human Ecology, Seoul National University, Seoul, Republic of Korea

J Nutr Biochem 2017;42:51–61

Background: Fetal growth and development are known to be affected by the In utero environment. More specifically, in offspring exposed to soy protein isolate (SPI) or genistein, a distinct fetal programming of carcinogenesis was reported.

Aims: The aim of the current study was to investigate whether hepatic gene expression and liver development of rat offspring is altered by maternal consumption of low-isoflavone SPI or genistein.

Methods: A 3-arms interventional study was conducted. Female Sprague-Dawley rats were fed a casein diet, a low-isoflavone SPI diet or a casein diet supplemented with genistein (250 mg/kg diet) for two weeks before mating and throughout pregnancy and lactation. Male offsprings were studied on postnatal day 21 (CAS, SPI and GEN groups).

Results: Among 965 differentially expressed hepatic genes related to maternal diet (P≤.05), a significantly different expression of 590 was found between the CAS and SPI groups. When comparing the CAS and GEN groups, the expression of 88 genes was significantly different between the groups. This difference mainly involved genes related to drug metabolism that were significantly affected by maternal diet.

Conclusions: Maternal consumption of a low-isoflavone SPI diet alters the hepatic gene expression profile and liver development in offspring possibly by epigenetic processes.

Comments   Data from both human and animal studies indicate that maternal nutrition and other environmental factors can alter the in utero development, which may further result in changes in the offspring susceptibility of chronic disease later in life. These modifications have been proposed to occur by altering epigenetic state of the fetal genome, such as DNA methylation and post-translational histone modification, caused by maternal nutrition.

The current study was aimed to determine whether maternal consumption of a low-isoflavone SPI diet and a casein diet supplemented with genistein could alter the hepatic gene expression and liver development in rat offspring. Despite the fact that previous studies have demonstrated the effect of maternal diet on the development of metabolic disease in the offspring, the use of gene expression profiling in a specific organ of young offspring was not extensively studied before.

The results of the current study suggest that the hepatic gene expression may be altered by amino acid composition or other bioactive components of SPI rather than soy isoflavone per se. An increased cell proliferation, reduced apoptosis, and activation of the mTOR pathway were shown in the SPI group. This may have contributed to a higher relative liver weight compared to other groups. In addition, the researchers observed higher serum homocysteine levels and lower global and CpG site-specific DNA methylation of Gadd45b, a gene involved in cell proliferation and apoptosis, in SPI group compared to CAS group.

These observations are not only interesting, but also important. We believe that in the era of extensive gene research, more studies assessing the influence of maternal diet on neonatal gene expression (in different end organs) should be performed to support studies addressing only clinical parameters.

Overall commentary

Adiposity and its related comorbidities has become prevalent worldwide, with the World Health Organization estimating that over 40 million children aged under 5 years are obese. There is no single method to define neonatal adiposity. Therefore, in the current chapter, novel studies addressing this issue in various perspectives were presented and discussed. Although maintaining a balanced maternal diet may improve offspring outcome, the impact of nutrition on fetal/offspring growth and development is also attenuated by genetic, demographic, behavioral, and other factors. Thus, maternal nutrition, like any other intervention, should be personalized to achieve its maximal benefit.

Disclosure Statement

The authors report no conflict of interest.

References

1 Pérez-López FR, Pasupuleti V, Mezones-Holguin E, et al: Effect of vitamin D supplementation during pregnancy on maternal and neonatal outcomes: a systematic review and meta-analysis of randomized controlled trials. Fertil Steril 2015;103:1278–1288.e4.

2 De-Regil LM, Palacios C, Lombardo LK, et al: Vitamin D supplementation for women during pregnancy. Cochrane Database Syst Rev 2012;2:CD008873.

Koletzko B, Shamir R, Turck D, Phillip M (eds): Nutrition and Growth: Yearbook 2018.
World Rev Nutr Diet. Basel, Karger, 2018, vol 117, pp 165–175 (DOI: 10.1159/000484505)

Stunting in Developing Countries

Andrew M. Prentice

Nutrition Theme, MRC Unit The Gambia, Fajara, Gambia

Introduction

Although stunting rates in low- and middle-income countries have been declining quite rapidly, with many countries meeting their Millennium Development Goal targets, there remain an estimated 160 million stunted children worldwide. As one of its Nutrition Targets, the World Health Organization (WHO) has set an ambitious goal of a further 40% reduction by 2025. Unfortunately, the rate of reduction in Africa is so slow that it is being more than offset by population growth such that the absolute numbers of stunted children is rising in this region.

In scanning all the papers published on this topic during the year under review, there is a depressing preponderance of descriptive papers that simply summarize the anthropometric statistics by region, country, area or population group with some of these papers including analyses of factors predictive of poor growth. The great problem with such analyses is that the factors associated with growth failure are all generally correlated with poverty and hence – apart from global eradication of poverty – it is hard to navigate through the statistical confounding and pinpoint individual factors that predispose to stunting. Some of these analyses do a much better job than others, and the examples are listed below.

Key articles reviewed for the chapter

Growth faltering in rural Gambian children after four decades of interventions: a retrospective cohort study

Nabwera HM, Fulford AJ, Moore SE, Prentice AM

Lancet Glob Health 2017; 5:e208–e216

Handwashing, sanitation and family planning practices are the strongest underlying determinants of child stunting in rural indigenous communities of Jharkhand and Odisha, Eastern India: a cross-sectional study

Saxton J, Rath S, Nair N, Gope R, Mahapatra R, Tripathy P, Prost A

Matern Child Nutr 2016; 12: 869–884

Impact of contaminated household environment on stunting in children aged 12–59 months in Burkina Faso

Fregonese F, Siekmans K, Kouanda S, Druetz T, Ly A, Diabaté S, Haddad S

J Epidemiol Community Health 2017; 71: 356–363

Female-headed households associated with lower childhood stunting across culturally diverse regions of Pakistan: results from a cross-sectional household survey

Khalid H, Martin EG

Matern Child Health J 2017; 21: 1967–1984

Risk factors for childhood stunting in 137 developing countries: a comparative risk assessment analysis at global, regional, and country levels

Danaei G, Andrews KG, Sudfeld CR, Fink G, McCoy DC, Peet E, Sania A, Smith Fawzi MC, Ezzati M, Fawzi WW

PLoS Med 2016; 13:e1002164

Environmental enteric dysfunction and growth failure/stunting in global child health

Owino V, Ahmed T, Freemark M, Kelly P, Loy A, Manary M, Loechl C

Pediatrics 2016; 138:e20160641

Systemic inflammation, growth factors, and linear growth in the setting of infection and malnutrition

DeBoer MD, Scharf RJ, Leite AM, Férrer A, Havt A, Pinkerton R, Lima AA, Guerrant RL

Nutrition 2017; 33: 248–253

Causal pathways from enteropathogens to environmental enteropathy: findings from the MAL-ED birth cohort study

Kosek MN, et al; for the MAL-ED Network Investigators (159 collaborators)

EBioMedicine 2017; 18: 109–117

Eggs in early complementary feeding and child growth: a randomized controlled trial

Iannotti LL, Lutter CK, Stewart CP, Gallegos Riofrío CA, Malo C, Reinhart G, Palacios A, Karp C, Chapnick M, Cox K, Waters WF

Pediatrics 2017; 140:e20163459

Growth faltering in rural Gambian children after four decades of interventions: a retrospective cohort study

Nabwera HM[1,2], Fulford AJ[1,2], Moore SE[1,3], Prentice AM[1,2]

[1]MRC Unit The Gambia, Banjul, The Gambia; [2]MRC International Nutrition Group, London School of Hygiene and Tropical Medicine, London, UK; [3]Division of Women's Health, King's College London, London, UK

Lancet Glob Health 2017; 5:e208–e216

Background: Recent estimates suggest that the rate of stunting has declined in many regions. However, it has declined very slowly in sub-Sahara Africa. Due to this very slow decline in the prevalence of stunting, and the growth in population, the absolute number of children with stunting has increased. Thus, it is important to identify effective intervention methods.

Methods: This was a cohort study using routine growth monitoring data from birth to age 2 years of 3,659 children between 1976 and 2012. The authors analyzed the effect of 36 years of intensive health interventions on growth in infants and young children from three rural Gambian villages. Z scores for weight-for-age, length-for-age, weight-for-length, mid-upper-arm circumference, and head circumference were calculated using the World Health Organization 2006 growth standards. Seasonal patterns of mean Z scores were obtained by Fourier regression.

Findings: Secular improvements were noted in all postnatal growth parameters, except weight-for-length, accompanied by declines over time in seasonal variability. The proportion of children who were underweight or stunted at 2 years of age halved during four decades of the study period, from 38.7% (95% CI 33.5–44.0) for underweight and 57.1% (95% CI 51.9–62.4) for stunting. However, despite the unprecedented extent of intervention, postnatal growth faltering persisted, leading to poor nutritional status at 24 months.

Interpretation: A combination of nutrition-sensitive and nutrition-specific interventions has caused a reduction of 50% in undernutrition rates. Yet, considerable growth faltering remains. It is important to learn and understand the causes to growth faltering to be able to develop new interventions.

Handwashing, sanitation and family planning practices are the strongest underlying determinants of child stunting in rural indigenous communities of Jharkhand and Odisha, Eastern India: a cross-sectional study

Saxton J[1], Rath S[2], Nair N[2], Gope R[2], Mahapatra R[2], Tripathy P[2], Prost A[1]

[1]UCL Institute for Global Health, London, UK; [2]Ekjut, Chakradharpur, Jharkhand, India

Matern Child Nutr 2016; 12: 869–884

Introduction: The WHO is aiming to reduce by 40% the number of stunted children worldwide by 2025. Approximately 55 million children affected by stunting live in India, and children from poorest families from Scheduled Caste and Scheduled Tribe communities are the worst affected.

The aim of the study was to identify the strongest factors causing stunting among these children in rural Jharkhand and Odisha in India to find the most relevant intervention methods.

Data were collected in 2010 from 1,227 children aged 6 months to 3 years and their mothers, from 18 clusters of villages in 3 districts with a high proportion of people from the "depressed classes." The authors measured height and weight of mothers and children, and captured data on various basic, underlying and immediate determinants of undernutrition. Generalized Estimating Equations were used to identify individual determinants associated with children's height-for-age z-score (HAZ; $p < 0.10$); the authors included these in a multivariable model to identify the strongest HAZ determinants using backwards stepwise methods.

In the adjusted model, the strongest protective factors for linear growth included cooking outdoors rather than indoors (HAZ +0.66), birth spacing ≥24 months (HAZ +0.40), and handwashing with a cleansing agent (HAZ +0.32). The strongest risk factors were later birth order (HAZ −0.38) and repeated diarrhoeal infection (HAZ −0.23). The results suggest multiple risk factors for linear growth faltering in indigenous communities in Jharkhand and Odisha. Interventions that could improve children's growth include reducing exposure to indoor air pollution, increasing access to family planning, reducing diarrhoeal infections, improving handwashing practices, increasing access to income, and strengthening health and sanitation infrastructure.

Impact of contaminated household environment on stunting in children aged 12–59 months in Burkina Faso

Fregonese F[1], Siekmans K[2], Kouanda S[3], Druetz T[1], Ly A[3, 4], Diabaté S[4], Haddad S[4]

[1]Centre de Recherche du CHUM (CRCHUM), Études de populations, Montréal, Québec, Canada; [2]HealthBridge, Ottawa, Ontario, Canada; [3]Institut de Recherche en Sciences de la Santé (IRSS), Ouagadougou, Burkina Faso; [4]Centre de Recherche du Centre Hospitalier Universitaire de Québec, Hôpital Saint-Sacrement, Montréal, Québec, Canada

J Epidemiol Community Health 2017; 71: 356–363

Background: One hundred sixty-five million children worldwide suffer from stunting, which affects their survival and development. Increasing evidence suggests that environmental enteropathy disorder (EED) may play a significant role in children with faltering growth, with a likely contribution of frequent fecal-oral transmission.

Aim: The aim of this study was to assess the impact of fecal-oral transmission on stunting in Burkina Faso, where stunting prevalence is very high.

Methods: Data were collected from a household panel study that was set up in 2011 as part of the Kaya Health and Demographic Surveillance System. Cohort consisted of children aged 1–5 years in Kaya. Data on household socioeconomic characteristics, food needs, and environmental contamination were collected once, and child growth parameters were measured annually, between 2011 and 2014. The authors used multiple correspondence analysis and 12 questions and observations on water, sanitation, hygiene behaviors, yard cleanliness, and animal proximity, to construct a "contaminated environment" index as a measure of exposure to fecal-oral transmission. Analysis was performed using a generalized structural equation model, adjusting for repeat observations and hierarchical data.

Results: Stunting (<2 SD height-for-age) was found in 29% of 3,121 children (median [interquartile range] age 36 [25–48] months). Environment contamination was highly prevalent, especially in rural and peri-urban areas, and was positively correlated with stunting (prevalence ratio 1.30; $p = 0.008$), after controlling for sex, age, survey year, setting, mother's education, father's occupation, household food security, and wealth. This association was significant for children of all ages (1–5 years) and settings. The effect of lower contamination was comparable to that of higher food security.

Conclusion: This study suggests that environment contamination may play an important part in the pathogenesis of stunting. Interventional programs for prevention of stunting should aim to reduce environmental contamination and fecal-oral transmission.

Female-headed households associated with lower childhood stunting across culturally diverse regions of Pakistan: results from a cross-sectional household survey

Khalid H[1], Martin EG[1, 2]

[1]Rockefeller College of Public Affairs and Policy, University at Albany-State University of New York, Albany, NY, USA; [2]Rockefeller Institute of Government, State University of New York, Albany, NY, USA

Matern Child Health J 2017; 21: 1967–1984

Objectives: The focus on female empowerment created interest in studying how it can also improve child health outcomes, and literature on this topic is plentiful. However, very little has been studied on the relationship between female empowerment and childhood stunting. Early childhood stunting has an adverse effect on long-term cognitive and health outcomes. The authors, therefore, explored this relationship among young children in Punjab, Pakistan, which has both high stunting rates and a considerable proportion of female-headed households. They also tried to assess whether this relationship varied within three provincial regions with differing cultural attitudes towards women's role in society.

Methods: The authors collected data from a cross-sectional household level survey performed in 2011, identifying 13,412 children aged 1–4 from 8,985 two-parent households in three culturally distinct regions in Punjab. Logistic regression models were used to estimate whether stunting was associated with female-headed households, as a reflection of female empowerment, and whether this relationship varied by region. Regressions were controlled for child- and household-level covariates.

Results: Children from female-headed households had 26% lower odds of stunting than children from male-headed households (OR 0.74, 95% CI 0.60–0.90). The interaction term for female-headed households and child stunting by provincial region was not statistically significant, suggesting that the relationship is valid across the three culturally distinct regions.

Conclusions: The results of this study suggest that women can improve child outcomes even after adjusting for access to medical care. Moreover, the results showed that with increased level of education for the household head, there is a reduction of stunting among children. Therefore, greater investments in public education and awareness campaigns to improve health literacy are needed for improving the success of existing public health interventions targeting childhood stunting.

Risk factors for childhood stunting in 137 developing countries: a comparative risk assessment analysis at global, regional, and country levels

Danaei G[1, 2], Andrews KG[1], Sudfeld CR[1], Fink G[1], McCoy DC[3], Peet E[1, 4], Sania A[1], Smith Fawzi MC[5], Ezzati M[6, 7], Fawzi WW[1, 2, 8]

[1]Department of Global Health and Population, Harvard T.H. Chan School of Public Health, Boston, MA, USA; [2]Department of Epidemiology, Harvard T.H. Chan School of Public Health, Boston, MA, USA; [3]Harvard Graduate School of Education, Cambridge, MA, USA; [4]RAND Corporation, Pittsburgh, PA, USA; [5]Department of Global Health and Social Medicine, Harvard Medical School, Boston, MA, USA; [6]MRC-PHE Centre for Environment and Health, School of Public Health, Imperial College London, London, UK; [7]Wellcome Trust Centre for Global Health Research, Imperial College London, London, UK; [8]Department of Nutrition, Harvard T.H. Chan School of Public Health, Boston, MA, USA

PLoS Med 2016; 13:e1002164

Background: Many risk factors for stunting have been identified in epidemiological studies, but their relative impact on stunting across developing countries is not known. This study aimed to evaluate the number of stunting cases in children aged 24–35 months and their relationship to 18 risk factors in 137 developing countries.

Methods and Findings: Risk factors were classified into five clusters: maternal nutrition and infection, teenage motherhood and short birth intervals, fetal growth restriction (FGR) and preterm birth, child nutrition and infection, and environmental factors. The authors derived the prevalence of exposure to each risk factor for the year 2010 from published literature and other available surveys, and estimated the prevalence of stunting and the number of stunting cases that were attributable to each risk factor and cluster by country and region. The leading risk factor across all countries studied was FGR (children born at term and small for gestational age), with 10.8 million cases (95% CI 9.1–12.6 million) of stunting (out of 44.1 million). The next most influential factors were unimproved sanitation, with 7.2 million (95% CI 6.3–8.2 million), and diarrhea with 5.8 million (95% CI 2.4–9.2 million). FGR and preterm birth was the leading risk factor cluster in all regions. Environmental risks had the second largest estimated impact on stunting globally and in the developing regions, whereas child nutrition and infection were the second leading cluster of risk factors in other regions.

The analysis is limited to risk factors for which data were available, and also required various approximations and assumptions.

Conclusions: This study found that FGR, unimproved sanitation, and diarrhea are the leading risk factors for stunting globally, with a bigger impact on stunting in developed regions than in other regions. Reducing the burden of stunting requires not only treatment of the affected infants, but also interventions focused on improving nutrition and sanitation for mothers and families.

Comments	The first paper by Nabwera et al. [1] sets the scene for what follows. It describes a 40-year longitudinal analysis of growth data collected in 3 rural Gambian villages that have benefitted from an unprecedented level of health interventions. There is good news and bad news. The good news is that stunting levels in 2-year olds were halved from 57 to 30%. The bad news is that despite the intense interventions that have had a profound effect on mortality, there is still a 30% rate of child stunting. This suggests that there is a very high threshold for interventions before stunting will be eliminated. What do these interventions consist of? This is where we need robust data on the primary etiological factors. The analysis by Saxton et al. [2] using data from Eastern India observed effect size associations that are unusually strong for this type of study. The strongest protective factors for linear growth included cooking outdoors rather than indoors (HAZ +0.66),

birth spacing ≥24 months (HAZ +0.40), and handwashing with a cleansing agent (HAZ +0.32). The strongest risk factors were later birth order (HAZ –0.38) and repeated diarrheal infection (HAZ –0.23).

A somewhat similar study in Burkino Faso attributed stunting to environmental contamination with a prevalence ratio of 1.30 in rural and peri-urban settings after adjusting for the measured potential confounders. As mentioned above there remains a risk of residual confounding in all such studies and the prevalence ratio of 1.3 is not very large. Thus, this and similar studies confirm what we already know about the relationship between poverty, living conditions and stunting, but do not give granular insights.

Khalid and Martin's study in Pakistan based on an analysis of household surveys showed that the risk of stunting was 24% lower in female-headed houses; from which they concluded that female empowerment and health literacy would be a good investment.

The final paper by Danaei et al. [3] offers a complex analysis of the impact of 5 clusters of risk factors for stunting in 137 developing countries. The authors acknowledge the limitations of their approach and stress that it only includes factors for which they could find published effect sizes. Nonetheless, they concluded that the leading risk worldwide was FGR, defined as being term and small for gestational age, with 10.8 million cases of stunting attributable to it (about one quarter of the total burden). This was followed by unimproved sanitation, with 7.2 million, and diarrhea with 5.8 million. FGR and preterm birth was the leading risk factor cluster in all regions. Environmental risks had the second largest estimated impact on stunting globally and in the South Asia, sub-Saharan Africa, and East Asia and Pacific regions, whereas child nutrition and infection were the second leading cluster of risk factors in other regions.

The next 3 papers relate to the long-discussed issue of how, and to what extent, EED lie on the causal pathway to stunting. This has been a topic of keen enquiry since the first demonstrations of chronic gut damage in young children in our own and other laboratories well over a quarter of a century ago.

Environmental enteric dysfunction and growth failure/stunting in global child health

Owino V[1], Ahmed T[2], Freemark M[3], Kelly P[4, 5], Loy A[6], Manary M[7], Loechl C[1]

[1]International Atomic Energy Agency, Vienna, Austria; [2]International Centre for Diarrhoeal Research, Bangladesh, Dhaka, Bangladesh; [3]Division of Pediatric Endocrinology, Duke University Medical Center, Durham, NC, USA; [4]University of Zambia, Lusaka, Zambia; [5]Blizard Institute, Queen Mary University of London, London, UK; [6]Department of Microbiology and Ecosystem Science, Research Network "Chemistry meets Microbiology," University of Vienna, Vienna, Austria; [7]Washington University, St Louis, MO, USA

Pediatrics 2016; 138:e20160641

Approximately 25% of the world's children aged <5 years suffer from stunting, which is associated with increased mortality, cognitive dysfunction, and loss of productivity. The global target is a 40% reduction in the number of stunted children by 2030. The pathogenesis of stunting is not fully understood. EED – a generalized disorder of small intestinal structure, commonly found in children living in unsanitary conditions – has a significant role in stunting. Mechanisms leading to growth failure in EED include increased intestinal permeability, gut inflammation, dysbiosis and bacterial translocation, systemic inflammation, and nutrient malabsorption. Since many causal pathways lead to EED, there is a need for versatile ways to treat it. Potential interventions to reduce EED include: (1) improved water, sanitation, and hygiene; (2) promotion of breastfeeding and diverse complementary nutrition; (3) probiotics and prebiotics; (4) nutrient supplements, including zinc, polyunsaturated fatty acids, and amino acids; (5) antiinflammatory agents such as 5-aminosalicyclic acid; and (6) antibiotics in the management of acute malnutrition and infection. Improved understanding of the events leading to EED and development of optimal diagnostic tools are still pending. "Omics" technologies (genomics, epigenomics, transcriptomics, proteomics, and metabolomics) and stable isotope techniques (e.g., ^{13}C breath tests) targeted at children and their intestinal microbiota may enhance our ability to successfully identify, manage, and prevent this disorder.

Systemic inflammation, growth factors, and linear growth in the setting of infection and malnutrition

DeBoer MD[1], Scharf RJ[2], Leite AM[3], Férrer A[3], Havt A[3], Pinkerton R[4], Lima AA[3], Guerrant RL[4]

[1]Pediatric Endocrinology, Department of Pediatrics, University of Virginia, Charlottesville, VA, USA; [2]Developmental Pediatrics, Department of Pediatrics, University of Virginia, Charlottesville, VA, USA; [3]Institute of Biomedicine, Federal University of Ceará, Fortaleza, Brazil; [4]Center for Global Health, University of Virginia, Charlottesville, VA, USA

Nutrition 2017; 33: 248–253

Objective: Recurrent infections are associated with lower growth velocity and stunting in children in developing areas of the world where malnutrition and recurrent infections are common. It is well known that both inflammation and malnutrition can result in growth hormone (GH) resistance, however, the interplay between infection, inflammation, and stunted growth in developing areas is not fully understood.

Aims: This study aimed to assess relationships between mild systemic inflammation, growth factors, and anthropometric measures in a case-control cohort of underweight and normal weight children in northern Brazil. The authors' hypothesis was that even low-grade inflammation would be associated with GH resistance, including lower levels of insulin-like growth factor-1 (IGF-1) and IGF-binding protein-3 (IGFBP-3) and higher levels of GH through lack of feedback.

Methods: Data from 147 children ages 6–24 months – evaluated in the MAL-ED case-control study – was assessed following recruitment from a nutrition clinic for impoverished families in Fortaleza, Brazil. Nonparametric tests and linear regression were used to evaluate correlations between symptoms of infections (assessed by questionnaire), systemic inflammation (portrayed by high-sensitivity C-reactive protein [hsCRP]), the GH IGF-1 axis, anthropometric measures. All models were adjusted for age and sex.

Results: Children with recent symptoms of diarrhea, cough, and fever had higher hsCRP levels than children without symptoms; those with recent diarrhea and fever also had lower IGF-1 and higher GH levels. There was a positive association between stool myeloperoxidase and serum hsCR. In turn, hsCRP was positively associated with GH and negatively associated with IGF-1 and IGFBP-3, assumedly reflecting a state of GH resistance. Following adjustment for hsCRP, IGF-1 and IGFBP-3 were positively and GH was negatively associated with z scores for weight and height.

Conclusions: The authors found that even mild inflammation in a cohort of significant poverty may lead to decreased growth, and a state of resistance to GH.

Causal pathways from enteropathogens to environmental enteropathy: findings from the MAL-ED birth cohort study

Kosek MN, et al. for the MAL-ED Network Investigators (159 collaborators)

Department of International Health, Johns Hopkins Bloomberg School of Public Health, Baltimore, MD, USA

EBioMedicine 2017; 18: 109–117

Background: EED, a state of persistent immune activation and altered permeability stemming from frequent and recurrent enteric infections, has been suggested as a major determinant of growth deficits in children in low- and middle-income countries. A theory-driven systems model to assess pathways by which enteropathogens, gut permeability, and intestinal and systemic inflammation influence child growth was developed within the framework of the Etiology, Risk Factors and Interactions of Enteric Infections and Malnutrition and the Consequences for Child Health and Development (MAL-ED) birth cohort study.

Methods: Non-diarrheal stool samples (n = 22,846) from 1,253 children from multiple sites within 8 countries were analyzed for markers of gut inflammation, a panel of 40 enteropathogens and fecal concentrations of myeloperoxidase, alpha-1-antitrypsin, and neopterin. Markers of gut permeability – urinary lactulose:mannitol (L:M; n = 6,363) and plasma alpha-1-acid glycoprotein (n = 2,797) – as well as anthropometric measures were also measured in the same cohort. A specific temporal sampling design was used to evaluate proposed mechanistic pathways leading to stunting in children 0–2 years of age.

Findings: In this cohort, frequent enteric infections and high levels of both intestinal and systemic inflammation were found. Higher loads of enteropathogens, especially those known to be entero-invasive or causing mucosal disruption, were linked with increased levels of gut and systemic inflammation markers, and thus indirectly associated with reduced linear and ponderal growth. Evidence supporting the association with impaired linear growth was more robust for systemic inflammation than for gut inflammation, but apparently reduced ponderal growth was more strongly correlated with local than systemic inflammation.

Interpretation: The substantial quantity of empirical data contributing to this analysis supports the conceptual model of EED. The impact of EED on growth faltering in young children was small, but the different analyses performed supported the attribution of growth failure to asymptomatic enteric infections. The strongest evidence for EED was the association between enteropathogens and linear growth mediated via systemic inflammation.

Comments
The paper by Owino et al. [4] reviewed the current knowledge linking EED to stunting and suggested 6 categories of potential interventions. The following 2 papers are among the early results from the multi-centre MAL-ED study funded by the Bill and Melinda Gates Foundation.

DeBoer et al. [5] describe the results from one of the MAL-ED sites in Brazil. Their results confirm the known links between infections, gut damage and inflammation, and systemic inflammation. They also assessed the GH/IGF-1 axis and found evidence of GH resistance in children with raised levels of systemic inflammation.

The final paper by Kosek et al. [6] summarizes the integrated results from all the MAL-ED sites, and therefore represents a very important piece of work. They present a heroic analysis including multiple measures of enteropathogen load in non-diarrheal stools, biomarkers of intestinal permeability and inflammation, and of systemic inflammation, and related these to subsequent growth using acyclic modelling. Again, the findings supported the current thinking with respect to the interconnecting pathways from enteropathogens to EED to systemic inflammation and growth restriction. However, the authors noted that the effect sizes were much smaller than anticipated. This might be a consequence of the renowned imprecision of measures of gut function which will necessarily introduce a high degree of correlation dilution.

The final paper is selected because it had an unusually large effect for an intervention against stunting; achieved by the provision of an egg per day.

Eggs in early complementary feeding and child growth: a randomized controlled trial

Iannotti LL[1], Lutter CK[2], Stewart CP[3], Gallegos Riofrío CA[4], Malo C[4], Reinhart G[5], Palacios A[5], Karp C[4], Chapnick M[1], Cox K[1], Waters WF[4]

[1]Brown School, Institute for Public Health, Washington University in St Louis, St Louis, MO, USA; [2]School of Public Health, University of Maryland, College Park, MD, USA; [3]Department of Nutrition, University of California, Davis, Davis, CA, USA; [4]Institute for Research in Health and Nutrition, Universidad San Francisco de Quito, Quito, Pichincha, Ecuador; [5]The Mathile Institute for the Advancement of Human Nutrition, Dayton, OH, USA

Pediatrics 2017; 140:e20163459

This manuscript was also discussed in Chapter 7, pages 129–150.

Aim: The aim of this study was to assess whether early introduction of eggs – a simple, affordable, and available source of nutrients – during complementary feeding would improve the growth and development of children from a resource-poor population.

Methods: This was a randomized controlled trial conducted in Ecuador, in which children aged 6–9 months were randomly assigned to intervention (an egg per day for 6 months [n = 83]) and control (no intervention [n = 80]) groups. Both arms received messages encouraging them to take part in this project. Household visits were performed once a week to monitor morbidity symptoms, distribute eggs, and monitor egg intakes (for egg group only). Baseline and end-point outcome measures included anthropometry, dietary intake frequencies, and morbidity symptoms.

Results: No allergic reactions to the eggs were reported. Generalized linear regression modeling revealed that the egg supplementation increased length-for-age z score by 0.63 (95% CI 0.38–0.88) and weight-for-age z score by 0.61 (95% CI 0.45–0.77). Log-binomial models with robust Poisson demonstrated a 47% reduction in the rate of stunting (prevalence ratio [PR] 0.53; 95% CI 0.37–0.77) and a 74% reduction in the prevalence of underweight (PR 0.26; 95% CI 0.10–0.70). Compared with controls, children in the intervention group had higher dietary intakes of eggs (PR 1.57; 95% CI 1.28–1.92) and a reduced intake of sugar-sweetened foods (PR 0.71; 95% CI 0.51–0.97).

Conclusions: This study suggests that the early introduction of eggs significantly improves growth in young children. Given the relative accessibility of eggs, this intervention may help to meet the global target set by the WHO to reduce stunting by 40% by 2025.

Comments The egg intervention increased length-for-age z-score by 0.63 and reduced the prevalence of stunting by 47%. These are impressive results in comparison even against all of the LNS studies that have used a product specifically designed to enhance child growth (see last year's Year Book). The authors note that "Eggs are a complete food, safely packaged and arguably more accessible in resource-poor populations than other complementary foods, specifically fortified foods" and "Moving forward, there is a need for effectiveness studies to identify scalable strategies to increase egg availability and access to vulnerable households and promote eggs early in the complementary feeding period in different cultural contexts."

In next year's Year Book, I look forward to being able to summarize the long-awaited results from the Wash Benefits Trials (in Kenya and Bangladesh) and the SHINE Trial in Zimbabwe. Initial results have been presented at conferences but not yet as full papers.

Reference

1   Nabwera HM, Fulford AJ, Moore SE, Prentice AM: Growth faltering in rural Gambian children after four decades of interventions: a retrospective cohort study. Lancet Glob Health 2017;5:e208–e216.

2   Saxton J, Rath S, Nair N, Gope R, Mahapatra R, Tripathy P, Prost A: Handwashing, sanitation and family planning practices are the strongest underlying determinants of child stunting in rural indigenous communities of Jharkhand and Odisha, Eastern India: a cross-sectional study. Matern Child Nutr 2016; 12:869–884.

3   Danaei G, Andrews KG, Sudfeld CR, Fink G, McCoy DC, Peet E, Sania A, Smith Fawzi MC, Ezzati M, Fawzi WW: Comparative Risk Assessment Analysis at Global, Regional, and Country Levels. PLoS Med 2016;13:e1002164.

4   Owino V, Ahmed T, Freemark M, Kelly P, Loy A, Manary M, Loechl C: Environmental Enteric Dysfunction and Growth Failure/Stunting in Global Child Health. Pediatrics 2016;138:e20160641.

5   DeBoer MD, Scharf RJ, Leite AM, Férrer A, Havt A, Pinkerton R, Lima AA, Guerrant RL: Systemic inflammation, growth factors, and linear growth in the setting of infection and malnutrition. Nutrition 2017;33:248–253.

6   Kosek MN, MAL-ED Network Investigators: Causal pathways from enteropathogens to environmental enteropathy: findings from the MAL-ED birth cohort study. EBioMedicine 2017;18:109–117.

Author Index

Gosoniu, L. 46
Goto, T. 99
Grant, S. 75
Gray, A.R. 19
Greenhawt, M. 50
Griffiths, A.M. 87
Grimberg, A. 1
Grimshaw, K. 50
Grisham, T. 148
Groetch, M.E. 50
Groome, A. 54
Groopman, J.D. 132
Grote, V. 125
Guerra, A. 118
Guerrant, R.L. 79, 147, 172
Gupta, A.K. 55
Gupta, R. 50
Gupta, S. 55

Ha, E.-H. 72
Habib, M.A. 139
Haddad, S. 168
Hagen, C.P. 10
Hagopian, W.A. 48
Hammond, B.R. 82
Han, A. 153, 163
Hankard, R. 114
Hanna, M. 19
Hanson, C. 58
Hao, W. 70
Harefa, B. 76
Hartman, C. 84
Hauner, H. 73
Havt, A. 172
Hawkes, C. 1
Hazell, T.J. 32
Heath, A.M. 19
Heath, K.E. 11
Hecht, R. 146
Heinen, F. 73
Heltshe, S.L. 92
Henriksen, C. 106
Hermsdörfer, J. 73
Heron, J. 81
Herskovitz, R. 89
Herviou, M. 114
Heubi, J.E. 92
Heuck, C. 10
Heude, B. 71
Hibbeln, J.R. 81
Hidayati, N. 76

Hiersch, L. 151
Hillman, C.H. 82
Hilton, J. 93
Hofmeister, B. 50
Hojsak, I. 43, 52
Høl, P.J. 75
Holick, M.F. 142
Hosono, H. 11
Huang, B. 87
Huang, R.C. 125
Huhtala, H. 101
Hulst, J. 43
Hulst, J.M. 52
Hume, R. 60
Hummel, S. 48
Husby, S. 115
Hussain, I. 139
Hwa, V. 11
Hwang, J.B. 50
Hyams, J.S. 87

Iannotti, L.L. 138, 174
Ibrahim, N.R. 63
Ierodiakonou, D. 54
Indrio, F. 43, 52
Ingrand, P. 114
Investigators of the CF trial 55
Islamiyah, A. 76

Jaddoe, V.W. 23, 24, 119
Jain, V. 55
Jamka, M. 30
Janssens, E. 46
Jarrold, K. 54
Jasani, B. 44, 69
Jeszka, J. 30
John, C.C. 79
Johnson, W. 159
Jones, G. 58
Jones, M.B. 160
Jorge, A.A. 12
Jorge, A.A.L. 11
Júlíusson, P.B. 106
Juloski, J. 9
Junek, R. 93
Juszczak, E. 60
Juul, A. 10

Kaar, J. 153
Kaar, J.L. 18, 158
Kac, G. 81

Kahrs, C.R. 103
Kaic, Z. 9
Kakietek, J. 146
Kamycheva, E. 99
Karlsson, M. 100
Karp, C. 138, 174
Katz, Y. 50
Kaufmann, M. 58
Kaukinen, K. 101
Kehoe, S.H. 80
Keller, K.L. 35
Kelly, P. 171
Kennedy, T.S. 75
Kenny, L.C. 160
Khalid, H. 169
Khan, G.N. 139
Khan, M.S. 136
Khan, N.A. 82
Khatry, S.K. 132
Kheng, T.H. 63
Kiefte-de Jong, J.C. 23, 24, 119
Kim, H. 72
Kim, Y. 72
Kivelä, L. 101
Kleinman, K. 142
Kloster, M. 92
Koletzko, B. 22, 125
Koletzko, S. 125
Konstantinou, G.N. 50
Korpela, K. 27
Kosek, M.N. 173
Koski, K.G. 117
Kouanda, S. 168
Kouwenhoven, S. 22
Kramer, A.F. 82
Kramer, M.S. 154
Krischer, J.P. 48
Krishna, A. 145
Krishnaveni, G.V. 80
Kroner, J. 97
Kuitunen, M. 27
Kukkonen, K. 27
Kull, I. 21
Kuran, M. 162
Kureishy, S. 139
Kurppa, K. 101
Kurtzman, T. 11
Kvammen, J.A. 106
Kwon, Y.H. 153, 163

Lafeber, H.N. 59

LaFranchi, S. 11
Lähdeaho, M.L. 101
Lalani, S. 11
Landberg, R. 29
Lapillonne, A. 43, 52
Larnkjær, A. 111, 115
Larsen, D.A. 148
Lass, N. 5
Lasschuijt, M. 35
Lauc, T. 9
Lauritzen, L. 29
Lawrence, J. 19
Lazar, A. 87
Lebl, J. 11
Lebovic, G. 31
Lee, E. 72
Lee, S.E. 132
Lee, Y.S. 26, 125, 154
Leite, A.M. 172
Lek, N. 26, 125
Leonard, M.B. 89
Leonard, S.A. 50
Leonardi-Bee, J. 54
Lernmark, A. 48
Leung, D.H. 92
Li, C. 117
Li, Y. 87
Lightdale, J. 50
Lima, A.A. 172
Lin, Y. 11
Lind, M.V. 111
Lindhardt Johansen, M. 10
Loechl, C. 171
Logan, A. 54
Longhi, S. 8
Lopes, C. 118
Los, E. 11
Loy, A. 171
Loy, S.L. 26, 125
Lum, J. 76
Lundin, K.E.A. 103
Lupi, F. 8
Lutter, C.K. 138, 174
Ly, A. 168
Lyden, E. 58

Ma, J. 156
Maalouf-Manasseh, Z. 136
Maas, C. 62
Magnus, M.C. 103
Magnusson, J. 21

Maguire, J.L. 31
Mahapatra, R. 167
Mäki, M. 101
Malkova, D. 140
Malo, C. 138, 174
Manary, M. 171
Martin, E.G. 169
Martorell, R. 70
Masarwi, M. 4
Massart, C. 6
Mathes, M. 62
Matias, S.L. 136
Mavromati, M. 6
Mazmanian, S.K. 78
Mazzanti, L. 8
McAuliffe, F.M. 157
McCowan, L.M.E. 160
McCoy, D.C. 170
McDonald, C. 96
McGhee, S. 50
McGovern, M.E. 145
McGrath, C.J. 134
McNaughton, S.A. 121
Mearin, M.L. 125
Mehr, S. 49, 50
Meldrum, S. 73
Mendez, M.A. 120
Meyer, R. 104
Miceli Sopo, S. 50
Michaelsen, K.F. 29, 115, 133
Michaelsen, K.F. 111
Mieritz, M.G. 10
Mihatsch, W.A. 43
Milasin, J. 9
Miller, J.D. 141
Millet, C. 114
Mis, N.F. 43, 52
Molgaard, C. 43, 52
Mølgaard, C. 111, 115
Moll, H.A. 23
Moller, M. 156
Monti, G. 50
Moore, S.E. 159, 167
Moradi, T. 21
Moreno, L.A. 15
Mori, T.A. 125
Moulton, C.J. 82
Mourath, D. 160
Mridha, M.K. 136
Muadz, H. 76
Muraro, A. 50

Nabwera, H.M. 167
Nair, N. 167
Namusoke, H. 133
Narine, L. 148
Nasir, A. 63
Nelson, C.A. 147
Nelson III, C.A. 79
Neufeld, L.M. 70
Newbern, D. 11
Nightingale, S. 93
Nilsson, O. 11
Ninjin, B. 142
Noel, S.K. 50
Nomura, I. 50
Noone, S. 50
Norris, J.M. 48, 158
Nowak, C. 11
Nowak-Wegrzyn, A. 50
Nshe, P. 159
Nurmatov, U. 54

O'Brien, E.C. 157
O'Connor, D.L. 31
Oddy, W.H. 125
Ogston, S. 60
Oliveira, A. 118
Olson, M. 11
Ooi, C.Y. 93
O'Sullivan, E.J. 157
Owino, V. 171

Palacios, A. 138, 174
Pallo, B.C. 70
Parkin, P.C. 31
Patole, S.K. 44, 69
Patro, B. 22
Paul, V.K. 55
Pearson, R.M. 81
Pedersen, D. 115
Peet, E. 170
Pereira, P. 146
Peter, A. 62
Petersen, J.H. 10
Peyre, H. 71
Phillip, M. 1, 4, 143
Piketty, M.L. 6
Pinkerton, R. 172
Plovier, H. 135
Poets, C.F. 62
Pohl, J. 96
Popovic, J. 11

Subject Index

Functional magnetic resonance imaging (fMRI)
    food energy density response and body
        composition 35, 36
    unhealthy food clue studies 33, 34

Genistein, soy protein isolate studies of hepatic
    gene expression in rat 163, 164
GH, *see* Growth hormone
Growth hormone (GH)
    deficiency
        differential diagnosis 5
        replacement therapy 8, 9
    therapy in Turner syndrome 9, 10
GUSTO study 154, 155
Gut microbiota
    cognition studies 77, 78
    malnutrition impact 135, 136
    obesity studies 27, 28
    pregnancy diet effects in infants 156, 157

Healthy Start study 153, 154, 158, 159
Hepcidin, anti-TNF therapy effects in Crohn's
    disease 89, 90

IGF-I, *see* Insulin-like growth factor-I
Inflammation
    malnutrition, infection, inflammation, and
        growth factors 172
    vitamin D studies in obesity 30, 31
Insulin-like growth factor-I (IGF-I)
    immunoassay 6, 7
    periconception nutrition effects on fetal
        sheep muscle development and
        hormones in growth 162, 163
Iodine
    cow's milk protein allergy and iodine
        status 106, 107
    pregnancy supplementation and cognition
        outcomes 74
    supplementation study in preterm
        infants 60, 61
Iron
    cognition outcomes after pregnancy 75–77
    formula fortification for young
        children 56–58
    inflammatory bowel disease iron deficiency
        anemia correction with iron
        sucrose 90–92

Leptin, milk composition in obese
    mothers 114, 115

Magnetic resonance imaging, *see* Functional
    magnetic resonance imaging
MAL-ED study 173, 174
Malnutrition
    biomarkers for risk stratification and
        intervention response 134, 135
    cognition impact 147
    complementary feeding egg studies 138,
        139, 174, 175
    egg study in Uganda school children 141,
        142
    environmental enteric dysfunction and
        growth failure 171–174
    female-headed household study of stunting
        in Pakistan 169
    Gambia stunting intervention
        evaluation 167
    gut microbiota impact 135, 136
    infection, inflammation, and growth
        factors 172
    intervention assessment in Pakistan 139,
        140
    investment framework for global reduction
        off stunting 146, 147
    linear growth
        dietary component modulation 143, 144
        intervention impact after 2 years of
            age 144, 145
    lipid-based nutrient supplementation 136,
        137
    plasma proteome and anthropometric
        status in Nepalese school children 132,
        133
    risk factors for stunting across developing
        countries 170, 171
    RUTF versus liquid oral nutrition
        supplement study 140, 141
    stunting and economic impact 145
    thymus size and changes during
        malnutrition treatment 133, 134
    vitamin D supplementation and growth
        in Mongol school children 142,
        143
Maternal intake, *see* Pregnancy diet
Metabolic syndrome, school meal effects on
    markers 29, 30
Milk, *see also* breastfeeding; Formula
    breast milk composition impact
        free amino acids and associations with
            maternal anthropometry and infant
            growth 115, 116